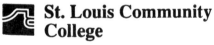

Pursuing Parenthood

Medical Ethics Series
David H. Smith and Robert M. Veatch, Editors

Pursuing Parenthood

ETHICAL ISSUES IN ASSISTED REPRODUCTION

Paul Lauritzen

INDIANA UNIVERSITY PRESS
Bloomington and Indianapolis

Parts of this work have appeared previously as "What Price Parenthood?" *Hastings Center Report* 20 (1990): 38–46; "Pursuing Parenthood: Reflections on Donor Insemination," *Second Opinion* 17/1 (1991): 57–76; and "'It Hain't the Money but the Principle o' the Thing': Some Problems for Surrogate Motherhood," Bloomington: The Poynter Center, 1991. The material appears here with permission.

The paper used in this publication meets the minimum requirements of American National Standard for Information Sciences—Permanence of Paper for Printed Library Materials, ANSI Z39.48-1984.

Manufactured in the United States of America

Library of Congress Cataloging-in-Publication Data

Lauritzen, Paul (Paul Joseph), date
Pursuing parenthood : ethical issues in assisted reproduction / Paul Lauritzen.
    p.   cm. — (Medical ethics series)
Includes bibliographical references and index.
ISBN 0-253-33261-3
1. Human reproductive technology—Moral and ethical aspects.
I. Title. II. Series.
RG133.5.L38 1993
176—dc20   92-16511

1 2 3 4 5   97 96 95 94 93

CONTENTS

ACKNOWLEDGMENTS

When I first decided to write about assisted reproduction I could not have imagined that a book would result. That one has is due largely to the support and encouragement of David H. Smith, who first convinced me that my initial reflections could be elaborated into a book-length study and then saw to it that they were. I am extremely grateful to him for his help and friendship as this project unfolded, and I am pleased as well to acknowledge the important contribution he made to the substance of the work. I am also pleased to offer special thanks to Lisa Sowle Cahill and Gilbert Meilaender, both of whom gave me the benefit of a very careful reading of large portions of the manuscript.

Although these three saved me from the largest number of mistakes, there are many others to whom I am also indebted for their suggestions or their friendship or both, including Adrienne Asch, Dena Davis, Rebecca Dresser, Howard Eilberg-Schwartz, Judy Granbois, Helen Bequaert Holmes, Kathryn Huey, Thomas E. Kelly, Jacqueline Lawson, Debra Marsey, Richard B. Miller, Thomas H. Murray, Louis Newman, Stephen Post, John P. Reeder, Jr., John Spencer, Robert Veatch, and Rosanne Zeidenweber.

I have also been fortunate to have had the opportunity to present parts of this work to various audiences and to benefit from their responses. My thanks go to the Center for Biomedical Ethics at Case Western Reserve University School of Medicine, Cleveland, Ohio; the Centre for Human Bioethics at Monash University, Melbourne, Australia; the Christian Centre for Bioethics, Sydney, Australia; the Poynter Center for the Study of Values and American Institutions, Indiana University, Bloomington, Indiana; and the Philosophy Department of Wooster College, Wooster, Ohio. The Alyce Vrolyk Institute for Bioethics, Northridge Hospital Medical Center; the Hastings Center; the Pacific Center for Health Policy and Ethics, University of Southern California; and the UniHealth America Bioethics Institute jointly sponsored a conference entitled "Families by Design," at which I was able to try out some of my ideas about assisted reproduction. I am grateful to the sponsors for the invitation to speak at this conference.

Even with all this help the book would not have been completed without the strong support of the administration at John Carroll University. Special thanks to Frederick F. Travis, Dean of the College of Arts and Sciences, and Sally Wertheim, Dean of the Graduate School, both of whom supported my research unreservedly. I have also had the extraordinary good fortune of working with a chairperson, Joseph F. Kelly, whose commitment to this work was steadfast, even when this commitment added to his own workload.

In doing the research for this book I relied heavily upon the good graces and efficiency of the librarians of Grasselli Library. Thanks to Bro. William Balconi, Ruth Reider, Mary Kay Sweeny, Caron Knapp, Nevin Mayer, Marcy Milota, and Chuck Zarobila. Two research assistants, Debra Marsey and Sheela Pawar, and two secretaries, Pam Waldschmidt and Mary Sharon Schumacher, made my life incalculably easier through their patience and skill.

The book was written during two leaves from teaching, one supported by a Grauel Faculty Fellowship from John Carroll University, the other supported by a N.E.H. Fellowship for college teachers. Both were indispensable to the successful completion of this project. For both I am profoundly grateful.

In many ways this is a book about the meaning of family. It is fitting, therefore, to conclude with a word of thanks to my own family, from whom I have learned so much about the meaning of the institution. Special thanks to my mother, Wilma Lauritzen, who has supported this project as she has so many other endeavors I have undertaken, that is to say, completely and unconditionally. Unconditional support from a parent is rare enough; to find it from the parents of one's spouse is truly exceptional. I am thus deeply grateful for the love and affection with which Frederick and Maria deFilippis welcomed me into their family. They thereby unwittingly taught me an important lesson about the nature of families. Thanks also to my sister-in-law, Diane Hayford and her spouse, Don Hayford, who have taught me a lot about what it means to be a parent, and to their children, Anne, David, and John, who have taught me that the bonds of affective kinship can be every bit as strong as those of genetic relation.

Finally, thanks to my spouse, Lisa deFilippis, with whom I have lived this book. What I owe to her cannot be measured; what I feel for her cannot be expressed. Thanks to her, my heart has not grown old.

The book is dedicated to my mother, Wilma Coffey Lauritzen, and to my son, Samuel Frederick Lauritzen, the two persons from whom I have learned the most about the meaning of parenthood.

INTRODUCTION

In the summer of 1985, my wife and I began what I now think of as our pursuit of parenthood. At the time, we certainly did not think about our attempt to conceive in anything like those terms; we were simply a married couple who had decided it was time to have children. Like many in our generation, we had postponed that decision for years as we each pursued graduate degrees. But by that summer I had completed my doctoral work, and Lisa had completed her penultimate year of law school. It seemed like a good point to begin a family. If we conceived in July or August, Lisa would be able to complete her final year of law school before the child was born. She might have to delay final examinations and thus graduation, but we had known other women who had done so without difficulty. She would certainly be unable to take the bar examination the following July, but we were willing to make the "sacrifice."

We did not conceive a child that July or August, nor would we for nearly four years. In retrospect, the combination of naïveté and romanticism with which we made our plans is embarrassing, if nothing else. Yet, at the time, we did not know that one in six couples in the United States is infertile; that perhaps as many as 1.2 million patients are treated annually for infertility-related problems; that approximately $1 billion are spent in the United States for infertility treatment every year.[1] Today, these are painful realities. By the time our child would have been born had our initial plans been realized, we had begun to suspect that we had a problem; six months later we were diagnosed as infertile and introduced to the world of high-tech reproductive medicine.

This book is about my encounter with that world. More specifically, it is about the moral questions raised—both for individual patients and for physicians—by current medical treatment for infertility and by currently available forms of assisted reproduction. When we began infertility treatment, the forms of assisted reproduction potentially available to us were made clear; the moral questions posed by these ways of having children were not. Artificial insemination with husband's sperm (AIH), *in vitro* fertilization (IVF), artificial insemination with donor sperm (DI), and adoption were all presented as options. Moreover, each was presented to us as simply one possibility among many: if one option failed to work, we could just turn to another. No significant medical distinctions were drawn among the various possibilities, nor was any suggestion made that we consider the morality of assisted reproduction.

In retrospect, this is puzzling, for each of the possibilities held out to us has been condemned as morally unacceptable by one group or another. Indeed, there is an extensive body of literature on the ethical questions raised by the new reproductive technology, much of it negative, and I will survey a fair amount of that literature in the chapters that follow. Regrettably, much of that work is abstract and unconnected to the actual experiences of individuals confronting reproductive decisions. Perhaps this should not be surprising, but I think it is troubling nonetheless. Of course, the fact that most opponents of reproductive technology have not directly experienced infertility treatment does not in any way invalidate the objections they raise. Still, there is a disturbing silence in contemporary discussions of assisted reproduction precisely where one would hope to hear an ongoing dialogue between those who condemn the coercion and degradation allegedly brought about by reproductive technology and those who are supposedly coerced and degraded. Instead, the voices of those who oppose reproductive technology but are fertile fail to reach, or are ignored by, the infertile on whose behalf these voices are often said to be raised. And the stories of those who are infertile and thankful for reproductive technology are unheard by those who too quickly and easily condemn this technology. This book is intended to break this silence by bringing together personal experience with infertility and theoretical reflection on the morality of assisted reproduction.

Many will ask why I would be willing to discuss the details of what is surely the most private of matters in a public forum. The answer is complex, but my essential motivation is born of the conviction that in reflecting on modern reproductive medicine we confront issues of profound importance. In this respect, I share Leon Kass's view that the issues raised by modern reproductive technology are not confined to questions of traditional medical ethics. Certainly we will need to ask of a procedure like IVF whether it necessarily violates accepted canons of medical ethics, but Kass is quite right to insist that we not overlook the broader questions raised by reproductive technology. As Kass writes, what is at stake is not just the "narrow issues of safety and informed consent" but the "*idea* of the *humanness* of our human life and the meaning of our embodiment, our sexual being, and our relation to ancestors and descendants."[2]

It is not just a conviction about the importance of the issues raised by the new reproductive technologies, however, that leads me to discuss my own experience. There is another reason grounded in a particular understanding of the role of concrete experience in moral reflection. In my view, all serious moral reflection must attend to the concrete experience of particular individuals and thus inevitably involves a kind of dialectical movement between general principles and our reactions to particular cases. The need to balance appeals to abstract rules and principles with attention to the affective responses of particular individuals has not always been sufficiently appreciated in moral theory or in medical ethics. Yet, as feminist writers (and others) have been insisting for some time now, such a balance is necessary if we are to understand both how moral decisions are actually made and how to act compassionately when faced with troubling moral decisions.[3]

Against the backdrop of these two convictions I offer my personal experience of infertility. I do not think that my experience is particularly unusual, but I do not doubt that others have had, or would have, very different experiences and would reach different conclusions. The fact that someone who is not a white heterosexual male might respond differently to the world of modern reproductive medicine does not vitiate the importance of appeals to concrete experience. To think that it does is to fail to understand that the dialectic between general principles and particular reactions is not a solipsistic movement. An appeal to personal experience is not a trump; it is not incorrigible; it is merely one item in a very long catalog of factors to be considered in trying to understand a given issue clearly. And the concrete experiences of others are among the items in that catalog.

Background

With these purposes in mind, then, let me provide a brief chronicle of my infertility treatment. This narrative will provide a context for some of the comments I will make later about assisted reproduction. As I have already hinted, our efforts to conceive a child were highly planned from the start. With careful deliberation, we planned the best time to have children given our two careers and were diligent in avoiding pregnancy until that time. What we had not anticipated was the possibility that pregnancy would not follow quickly once we stopped using birth control. This had not been the experience of our friends whose equally carefully laid plans had all been realized. For them, birth control ended and pregnancy followed shortly thereafter. For us, a year and a half of careful effort, including charting temperatures and cycles, yielded only frustration. We then sought professional help. A postcoital examination by my wife's gynecologist revealed few and rather immobile sperm. I was referred to a specialist for examination. As it turned out, I was diagnosed as having two unrelated problems: a varicocele and retrograde ejaculation. A varicocele is a varicose vein in the testicle that is sometimes associated with a reduction in both the numbers and quality of sperm. Retrograde ejaculation is a condition in which a muscle at the neck of the bladder does not contract sufficiently during ejaculation to prevent semen from entering the bladder. As a result of this condition, during intercourse semen is ejaculated into the bladder rather than into the vagina, as it would be under normal circumstances. Both conditions are treatable in many cases. Indeed, the doctor's diagnosis was followed almost immediately by a presentation of possible "therapies," given roughly in the order of the doctor's preferences, all presented as points on the same therapeutic continuum. A varicocele can be repaired surgically. Retrograde ejaculation can sometimes be eliminated through the use of drugs and, failing that, can be circumvented by recovering sperm from urine and using it for artificial insemination. Should both these treatments fail, *in vitro* fertilization might be successful; if IVF fails, donor insemination is a possibility. If none of these is successful, adoption can be pursued. Thus, at the start of treatment we were presented with a variety of options. Using drugs or surgery we could continue to try to conceive "naturally." Using artificial insemination or *in vitro* fertilization we could pursue parenthood with the available forms of assisted reproduction.

Since surgery for a varicocele is not always successful, and since surgery is more invasive than either of the treatments for retrograde ejaculation, I chose to address the latter problem first. Unfortunately, in my case, neither drug therapy nor artificial insemination was of any avail. Possibly because of damage done to the sperm as the result of the varicocele, the numbers and quality of sperm recovered from urine for insemination were not such to make conception likely. After trying artificial insemination for six months, we decided to attempt to repair the varicocele. Following surgery, there is generally a three- to nine-month period in which a patient can expect to see improvement in his sperm count. Nine months after my surgery there was virtually no improvement in either the numbers or the motility of the sperm. Although we resumed artificial insemination, the prospects were not good. After several unsuccessful attempts, our physicians advised us to consider *in vitro* fertilization, donor insemination, or adoption.

In honesty, we had reservations about each of these options. IVF is expensive, invasive, and generally not successful. Donor insemination is widely thought to be immoral and is certainly problematic emotionally. Adoption can be a long, expensive, and emotionally draining process. We decided to pursue *in vitro* fertilization, only to be told that, after further consideration of the numbers and quality of my sperm, we were not good candidates. This left donor insemination and adoption.

Because the process of adoption through an agency generally takes a minimum of two years, we had already decided to begin the process even if we continued infertility treatment. Thus, when *in vitro* fertilization was ruled out as an option, we knew already that we would pursue adoption, and we began the process shortly thereafter. We had only to decide whether to undertake donor insemination. This was certainly the hardest decision we confronted during our pursuit of parenthood, but ultimately we decided to go forward with DI.

Success rates with DI are very high, and when Lisa was not pregnant after several cycles, her physicians recommended a full infertility work-up for her. Since our adoption was moving along very smoothly at the time, we decided to forgo any additional infertility testing, and we focused all of our energies on collecting the large number of documents necessary for an international adoption. We scheduled and underwent the mandatory home study and awaited the social worker's report. In short, we had exhausted the resources reproductive medicine had to offer and consequently were planning to adopt. Nevertheless, we decided to continue infertility treatment until the report on our home study was complete and we could be placed on a waiting list of prospective adoptive parents. To our surprise and delight, we soon discovered that Lisa was pregnant.

This, in short, is the bare chronicle of my infertility experience. A complete record would be too personal, too painful, and too long to present here. But what exactly do I propose to examine in light of this experience? I will focus primarily on those forms of assisted reproduction that were made available to my wife and me. As I said, none of these options is free from controversy. Arguments have been vigorously pressed both in support of and in opposition to each of these reproductive technologies. In the chapters that follow, I will review some of the more compelling of these arguments. In considering the case for and against assisted reproduction, I will certainly attempt to do justice to the claims of both advocates and opponents considered in themselves. I will also at times want to ask whether the claims being made about some particular form of assisted reproduction find support in the lived reality of infertility treatment, at least as I experienced it.

Because this appeal to personal experience is rather unusual, let me try to explain more precisely how such appeals will function in what follows. There are primarily three ways in which I will make use of such considerations. The first and narrowest use has to do with the attempt to corroborate general claims made about reproductive technologies by asking whether such claims are in fact borne out in actual infertility treatment. Consider, for example, the claim often made by opponents of reproductive technology that the use of new techniques inevitably results in the treatment of human beings as products or commodities. Some feminists, for instance, have argued that reproductive medicine treats women as "living laboratories" in which body parts or systems are manipulated without sufficient knowledge about the consequences of such manipulation.[4] Others have claimed that assisted reproduction has broken down the process of procreation into the joining of discrete body parts which are, in theory, available for sale as commodities.[5] Still others have suggested that the obsessive pursuit of biological parenthood fueled by the new reproductive technologies results in an equally obsessive concern about the "quality" of the product, i.e., the child, manufactured by this technology.[6]

Although each of these claims can be evaluated independently of how individuals or couples experience infertility treatment, each nevertheless also has implications about the nature of such treatment that make appeals to experience relevant. If reproductive technology is indeed dehumanizing, if it results in the treatment of persons as products, if children are in fact reduced to products in its wake, then we should expect that at least reflective people undergoing infertility treatment will report feeling degraded, objectified, or excessively concerned about the "quality" of the children they seek. In other words, there ought to be at least some correspondence between the abstract claims made about the dangers of reproductive technology and the reports of those who are said to be at risk. Thus, I will suggest that in considering the claim that reproductive technologies lead, say, to the commodification of children, it is relevant to report that my wife and I found it very difficult to resist the goal-oriented "production" mentality that pervades infertility treatment. This fact alone does not, of course, establish the validity of the claims about the commodification of reproduction, but it does lend some support to the claim that, once procreation is separated from sexual intercourse, it is difficult not to treat procreation as the production of an object to which one has a right as the producer. This was certainly our experience: once we entered the world of reproductive medicine, it was difficult not to place the end above the means; effectiveness in accomplishing one's goals easily becomes the sole criterion by which decisions are made.

In suggesting that appeals to personal experience may serve a sort of corroborating function, I am also implying that the actual experience of treating for infertility may generate insights about assisted reproduction that are not easily accessible in other ways. This points to the second way in which attention to personal experience will be important to this volume. At a number of points I will rely on my own experience of infertility treatment to draw attention to features of assisted reproduction that would not be readily noticed from outside. Let me give an example. Although a number of writers have commented on the danger of coercion that arises with modern reproductive technology, these discussions have generally focused on two possible forms of coercion. Either attention is given to the social pressure placed on childless women to use reproductive technology in order to escape the stigma of childlessness, or attention is focused on a possible future in which women might be coerced to use reproductive technologies to diagnose and correct genetic defects.

Although these forms of coercion are worrisome and certainly need to be addressed, no one, so far as I know, has drawn attention to a third way in which reproductive technology may exert a sort of coercive pressure on infertile couples. Essentially, this pressure arises from the fact that the very existence of the technology inevitably changes the experience of infertility in ways that are not salutary. One of the peculiar aspects of infertility is that it is typically a condition that a couple suffers. As Leon Kass has noted, infertility is as much a relationship as a condition.[7] Yet infertility treatment, structured as it is by available technologies, leads us to view infertility individually. It is the individual who is treated, and it is the individual who must accept responsibility for childlessness, if he or she refuses treatment. From a situation in which infertility is a relational problem for which no one is to blame, infertility becomes an individual problem for which an individual who refuses treatment is to blame.[8]

This problem is compounded by the fact that infertility specialists simply assume that individuals will pursue all available treatments, and they typically present treatment options as just various points on the same therapeutic spectrum. These options are distinguished primarily by the degree of invasiveness of the respective treatment. In my case, taking relatively mild drugs in an effort to make an incontinent muscle more efficient lies at one end of the continuum, at the other end of which lies IVF.[9] Surgery, I suppose, falls somewhere in the middle. As I pointed out above, however, at no time in my treatment did anyone suggest that there existed a difference in kind among treatments.[10] It was generally assumed that if one therapy failed, we would simply move on to the next. And that is the problem I'm addressing here. If the technology exists, the expectation is that it will be used. If surgery might repair the problem, even if the chances are not great, how can I not have surgery? If surgery and artificial insemination have not worked, but IVF might, how can I not try IVF? The very availability of the technology appears to exert a sort of tyrannical pressure to use it.

The third way, then, in which appeals to personal experience will function in this volume is analogous to the role played by "moral conceptions" and "moral sensibilities" in what John Rawls calls "reflective equilibrium."[11] Reflective equilibrium is a method of theory testing in ethics by virtue of which one seeks to arrive at a coherent moral scheme in which there is a fit among a set of moral principles, and one's considered moral judgments—which incorporate moral conceptions and moral sensibilities—considered in light of the best competing moral theories. As Rawls describes the process: "One tries to see how people would fit their various convictions [including convictions about particular acts and institutions] into one coherent scheme, each considered conviction whatever its level having a certain initial credibility. By dropping and revising some, by reformulating and expanding others, one supposes that a systematic organization can be found."[12] Because I am not interested in either offering or testing an ethical theory, much less a theory of justice, it would be misleading to suggest that I will make use of the method of reflective equilibrium in assessing modern reproductive medicine. Nevertheless, the sort of back-and-forth movement Rawls envisions between general moral principles and particular judgments as one seeks to reach reflective equilibrium about a moral theory provides a useful model for depicting how appeals to personal experience can fruitfully be used in this study.

Since Rawls is interested in the idea of reflective equilibrium primarily as a method of theory acceptance in ethics, this notion does not fully model the function of appeals to experience in the present volume. In considering individual reaction to particular cases of assisted reproduction and to normative and descriptive judgments about these cases, I am not attempting to test an ethical theory so much as I am attempting to "test" the particular normative and descriptive judgments themselves. Thus, I need to supplement the model of reflective equilibrium if I am to make clear how I intend to proceed.

Toward this end, I want briefly to sketch an account of how one ought to test particular normative judgments offered by the philosopher Morton White.[13] According to White, justification in ethics should be modeled on the epistemic holism that Quine and others have brought to justification in science. In this view, one does not test descriptive statements or beliefs individually; rather, one tests aggregates of statements or beliefs. Quine, for example, rejects the notion that individual beliefs can be tested by comparing them to reality, and he insists, instead, that we evaluate bodies of beliefs. For Quine, these bodies of beliefs give rise to predictions about what sensory experiences to expect under given circumstances. If these experiences are not realized under the appropriate circumstances, we may need to question the entire system, for it was the system or body of beliefs that generated the prediction, not just an individual belief. As is well known, in Quine's view, nothing in this testing procedure is immune to revision. We may decide that our experience was mistaken, but we may equally decide that what we took to be a "law" of nature is inaccurate or even that established canons of logic must be discarded. What we seek is a body of descriptive beliefs that may be used as a tool for organizing or linking sensory experiences. And we make adjustments within this body of beliefs if there are recalcitrant sensory experiences.

According to White, much the same view can be taken toward justification in ethics. Just as we do not test descriptive judgments individually or in isolation, neither do we test normative judgments that way. Rather, we test normative judgments in a "corporatistic" manner by attending both to the descriptive and moral beliefs that lead to a particular normative conclusion and to our moral reactions to that conclusion. If our reactions do not support the conclusion, then we find ourselves in a situation analogous to that in which a sensory experience has not confirmed the body of scientific beliefs that predicted a different sensory experience. We are thus led, says White, to seek a revision somewhere among the components of the body of beliefs that led to this conclusion.[14]

White provides a nice example to illustrate his point. "Suppose," he writes, "that a mother has taken the life of a fetus that she has been carrying, and suppose that we present the following arguments":

(1) Whoever takes the life of a human being does something that ought not to be done.
(2) The mother took the life of a fetus in her womb.
(3) Every living fetus in the womb of a human being is a human being.

Therefore,

(4) The mother took the life of a human being.

Therefore,

(5) The mother did something that ought not to be done.[15]

In White's view, justification in ethics is such that if we deny that the woman in this example did something that ought not to be done, then we may be led to question the entire set of beliefs—both normative and descriptive—that gave rise to the moral judgment stated in (5). In White's words, "We may amend or surrender a law of logic like that which gets us from (2) and (3) to (4); an ethical law like (1); or a descriptive statement like (2), (3), or (4)."[16] Moreover, as White makes clear, we may be led to deny (5) and thus to question (1)–(4) precisely on the basis of feelings we have about this case. Indeed, for White, the feelings of obligation we have in connection with particular normative judgments are analogous to the sensory experiences that play so important a role in the justification of descriptive judgments in science. Just as we may be led to revise some body of descriptive beliefs because, say, a particular powder is not white, as we predicted it would be, so we may be led to revise our normative judgments about particular cases if our feelings reject the conclusions we have reached.[17]

That our emotions should be given such a prominent place in moral deliberation will strike some as mistaken; that they should be allowed to influence our description of the world will seem to many simply absurd. Yet this is what White means to suggest and, in many ways, I want to follow this suggestion in my appeals to personal experience in the chapters that follow. It seems to me that traditional moral theory has not paid sufficient attention to the role of what Bernard Williams has called "spontaneous convictions" in moral deliberation.[18] By spontaneous conviction I mean the untheorized and often passionate responses we have to particular moral issues.[19] When my students routinely reject Michael Tooley's well-known defense of infanticide, they often do so, at least initially, because they are emotionally repulsed by the prospect of killing an infant. This repulsion is their spontaneous conviction about infanticide. Tooley dismisses such a response as merely "visceral"—akin, he says, "to the reaction of previous generations to masturbation or oral sex."[20] Yet I see no reason to dismiss such responses so quickly.[21] On the contrary, I agree with White that we must take our spontaneous convictions seriously and that they may indeed lead us to rethink either a particular normative judgment or a line of argument leading to a particular moral judgment or both.

Thus, when I consider the morality of various forms of assisted reproduction, I will frequently appeal to my spontaneous convictions about the issues under consideration. In doing so, however, I want to emphasize once again that an appeal to a spontaneous conviction is the beginning, not the end, of a sustained discussion that may ultimately result in the revision of a normative judgment, a descriptive judgment, or the spontaneous conviction itself. As H. Tristram Engelhardt, Jr., has pointed out, "One often discovers, with chagrin, that one's most heartfelt convictions are indefensible prejudices."[22] So Tooley may indeed be right that our abhorrence of infanticide is like a previous generation's disgust at masturbation, but he may be wrong, too.

The important point is that our initial abhorrence of infanticide may drive us to reconsider Tooley's argument about the nature of personhood because we feel that he cannot but be wrong and thus our initial response plays a critical role in moral deliberation. In a similar vein, I suggest that the spontaneous convictions of those who have undergone infertility treatment may lead us to reconsider many of the claims that have been made about forms of assisted reproduction. Many have argued, for example, that donor insemination is morally problematic because it is a form of adultery. Yet my own experience suggests that, whatever problems may beset donor insemination, this is surely not one of them. In other words, my spontaneous conviction about the claim that donor insemination is a form of adultery is that such a claim is badly mistaken and that we must return to the body of beliefs and reasoning that produced that judgment in order to see where a mistake has been made.

To summarize, then, I appeal to personal experience or what I have just called spontaneous conviction in three ways. First, I seek to corroborate claims made about the impact of reproductive technologies on those who avail themselves of them. Second, I draw attention to aspects of assisted reproduction that are most easily appreciated from inside the world of modern reproductive medicine. Third, I make use of personal experience as part of a dialectical process of moral deliberation in which one seeks a sort of equilibrium among normative principles and descriptive beliefs, particular normative judgments and spontaneous convictions, including emotions.

The study itself is divided into three parts and is organized roughly around the specific forms of assisted reproduction that were made available to us. In the first chapter, I take up what is probably the least controversial form of assisted reproduction, artificial insemination with husband's sperm. Although there appears to be a general consensus in our society that AIH is morally acceptable, the Catholic church has censured AIH as a morally inappropriate response to infertility. To identify the most basic opposition to assisted reproduction, I examine the Vatican *Instruction on Respect for Human Life in Its Origins and on the Dignity of Procreation*.[23] I argue that there are two bases for the Vatican's opposition, one rooted in a traditional act-oriented natural law approach to human sexuality and one rooted in a concern about an alleged dualism at the heart of reproductive technology that may lead us to treat persons as products. While I reject the argument from natural law, I suggest that there is much more to be said in favor of the Vatican's concern about dualism. Specifically, I claim that the disembodiment of procreation entailed by AIH is indeed dualistic and that the Vatican is legitimately concerned that such disembodied procreation can lead us to think of procreation as a mechanistic, technical enterprise, reducible to the joining of gametes.

This general concern about disembodied procreation is further explored in chapters 2 and 3, where I consider *in vitro* fertilization and its many applications. In chapter 2 I take up what I call the simplest case, namely, IVF within a marriage where care is taken to avoid destroying or risking embryos. Although many have opposed even this simplest application, I argue that the two principal objections to IVF narrowly considered are not sufficient to justify complete opposition to this technology. Nevertheless, when we turn in chapter 3 to consider application of IVF technology beyond the simplest case, we discover that the worries about the commodification and mechanization of reproduction introduced in chapter 1 become increasingly grave. The expansion of IVF technology beyond its original boundaries has initiated a process in which human procreation is frequently cast in the language of the marketplace. Yet if procreation is thereby reduced to a production process, the access to and control over human gametes made possible through *in vitro* fertilization may well lead to genetic engineering, as opponents of IVF have argued. If procreation is indeed treated on the model of production, the attraction of genetic engineering will be obvious: genetic screening and therapy would be a sort of quality control mechanism in the manufacturing process.

Although the first three chapters raise concerns about AIH and IVF, and although I suggest that we move cautiously as a society in embracing these forms of assisted reproduction, in general I affirm both procedures as morally acceptable responses to infertility. In short, I try to show why the basic opposition to reproductive technology is misplaced. Perhaps inevitably, the discussion in these first three chapters is largely reactive. By contrast, in part II, I attempt to offer a more positive and constructive position on the morality of assisted reproduction by taking up the question of what it means to be a parent. I ask this question in chapter 4 by turning to consider applications of artificial insemination and *in vitro* fertilization that many find morally objectionable. Specifically, I take up artificial insemination with donor sperm and *in vitro* fertilization with donor eggs. Many who accept AIH and IVF when donor gametes are not used draw the line when assisted reproduction involves third parties donating gametes. This chapter explores the question of whether dividing up genetic, gestational, and social parenthood is intrinsically morally problematic. I examine a variety of arguments that support the importance of keeping genetic and social parenthood together, but ultimately I suggest that dividing genetic and social parenthood is not wrong. In other words, I suggest that drawing the boundary between morally acceptable and morally unacceptable forms of assisted reproduction in a way that insists on keeping genetic and social parenthood together is not salutary and that we would be better served in our line drawing by being responsive to social relationships rather than to genetic ties.

In chapter 5 I suggest that if we are responsive to social relationships rather than to genetic ties, we will not lump together surrogate motherhood and donor insemination, as is so often done in the literature on surrogacy. Since surrogate motherhood is a form of assisted reproduction that addresses infertility in women, this was not a reproductive option that my wife and I directly confronted. Nevertheless, I take up surrogacy because so many writers have compared it to donor insemination and have argued that, if DI is morally acceptable, so, too, is surrogacy. The suggestion is that advocates of DI are, at least implicitly, advocates of surrogacy. I show in chapter 5 why this is not the case. As we explore the differences between DI and surrogacy, we will come to see more clearly why it is important to attend to the concrete social relationship between parent and child rather than to abstractions like "genetic connection."

Finally, in part III, I discuss the alternative to reproductive technology endorsed by most opponents of assisted reproduction, namely, adoption. The final chapter thus concerns the morality of adoption. Although adoption is not really a form of assisted reproduction, it is important to consider because it is so frequently held out to be a better alternative for infertile couples than the resort to reproductive technology. In other words, critics of reproductive technology often point to the potential difficulties associated with IVF or DI or surrogacy and then ask how undertaking these procedures can possibly be justified when a childless couple could adopt, thereby avoiding these difficulties and helping a parentless child. Unfortunately, such comparisons often assume that adoption is morally unproblematic. I argue that adoption is not as unproblematic as it first appears. When we look at current adoption practice, we see some of the same dangers found in reproductive medicine. In the trend toward independent and international adoptions we see a shift toward commercialization. Indeed, as it is sometimes practiced in this country, it is difficult to consider adoption as anything other than the purchase of a product. Adoption may also involve a substitution of one form of coercion for another: a woman who feels she must have a child in order to be whole takes the child of a woman who feels she has no choice but to give up a child. I conclude that adoption is not the panacea that critics of reproductive technology often assume.

If I had to summarize the view of assisted reproduction developed in the pages below, I would describe it as guarded approval. That my basic position is one of qualified endorsement will be evident from the fact that, of the various general forms of assisted reproduction which I consider in this volume, commercial surrogate motherhood is the only one that I argue cannot be morally justified. For many critics of reproductive technology, such a conclusion will render any criticisms I raise ultimately innocuous. Indeed, one person who read earlier versions of this work remarked that my guarded approval reminded him of Paul Ramsey's comment about a similarly moderate approach to abortion: "ample abortions, always with tears."[24] Although I understand how my reservations about assisted reproduction might be construed in this fainthearted fashion, I do not mean to say that every use of assisted reproduction is morally defensible, so long as it is accompanied by enough hand-wringing. To say that IVF or DI can be justified morally is not to say that IVF or DI is always justified. For example, when I say that donor insemination as it is currently practiced is flawed because of the secrecy that surrounds it, but that in general DI can be justified, I do not mean that DI undertaken in secret is acceptable, provided that the participants agonize over the secrecy. Rather, I mean that DI undertaken in secret is morally unacceptable. If my reservations are infrequently framed in the language of condemnation, it is—as with so much in this volume—partly because of my experience. I have experienced the profound joy and fulfillment of having a child. Consequently, I am reluctant to judge the actions of those who seek what I have been so blessed to have received, even when they seek such a good in ways that I believe are fundamentally misguided.

Part I

Basic Opposition to Reproductive Technology

1

Dualism and Disembodiment?

The Case of AIH

Discussions of assisted reproduction often begin and end with a consideration of the most controversial interventions in the reproductive process. So we should not be surprised to discover that much of the literature on the morality of assisted reproduction has concerned issues like *in vitro* fertilization and surrogate motherhood. As important as it is to come to grips with forms of reproductive technology that have generated significant public disagreement and about which there is little societal consensus, it is also important to be mindful that there is as much to be learned from quiet as from clamor. Indeed, the very fact that any form of intervention in the reproductive process is socially sanctioned is significant and reveals the importance of the values and interests at stake here. Moreover, choices about controversial interventions are not made in a vacuum; they emerge against a background in which a range of reproductive options are in view, including options that are considered to be perfectly acceptable. Someone deciding whether to pursue homologous *in vitro* fertilization is likely to frame the decision in terms of the surrounding reproductive choices: homologous IVF may seem like a reasonably desirable option when it is framed as perhaps more questionable than AIH but considerably less morally problematic than DI or surrogate motherhood.

I thus begin with a consideration of what is probably the least controversial form of assisted reproduction currently available: artificial insemination with husband's sperm. Since many decisions concerning reproductive interventions are made against the backdrop of a general acceptance of AIH, if we can clarify why this procedure is commonly believed to be unproblematic as well as why it is nevertheless thought by some to be deeply troubling, we will have made a good start in facing some of the disturbing questions raised by current reproductive medicine.

Basic Facts about AIH

Artificial insemination with husband's sperm is one of the most widely practiced reproductive interventions.[1] According to the Office of Technology Assessment, each year approximately 90,000 women undergo artificial insemination with their husband's sperm.[2] From this group, OTA estimates, 35,000 children are born annually. Why do so many women pursue artificial insemination, and why is AIH as socially acceptable as it appears to be?

The answers to these questions are related. AIH is one of the few available treatments for male-factor infertility, it is relatively noninvasive, and it is perhaps as close to the ideal of conceiving through natural sexual intercourse as any form of assisted reproduction can be. Consider the typical case of AIH. A couple who has been unable to conceive a child after a year of trying comes to an infertility specialist for a work-up. The tests show that, while the woman appears to be fertile, the man has a low sperm count or low sperm motility or is unable to deposit semen in his wife's reproductive tract. The doctor recommends artificial insemination with the husband's sperm and explains that this procedure will involve charting cycles to pinpoint ovulation, collecting semen through masturbation, preparing the semen for insemination, and depositing the collected semen in the woman's vagina or uterus through a catheter.

Given the simplicity of this procedure, it should not be surprising that large numbers of couples will choose to pursue this option when it is offered to them as the best hope they have of conceiving a child together. Nor should it surprise us that they will be supported in their decision by widespread social approval. As a society we clearly affirm the value of having children, and we acknowledge that the desire to reproduce is important and powerful. Indeed, the fulfillment of the desire to have children is often thought to be so basic to human flourishing that it is sometimes said to generate a right to procreate. The Supreme Court, for example, has repeatedly recognized such a right for married couples, at least implicitly.[3] Indeed, Justice White's review of the law in this regard, in *Stanley v. Illinois,* might well stand as a fair statement of general social views on the importance of reproduction. "The rights to conceive and to raise one's children," he says, "have been deemed 'essential.' " They are "basic civil rights of man" and are "far more precious . . . than property rights."[4]

Granting, then, that the desire to have children is socially sanctioned and that the procedure for AIH appears to be so simple and harmless, on what grounds could anyone oppose it? It is to this question that I wish to devote most of the rest of this chapter. In considering this question I turn to consider the two most sustained attacks on reproductive technology in the literature on assisted reproduction, one religious and one secular. I begin with an examination of the opposition raised to AIH by the Roman Catholic church, primarily as it is formulated in the *Instruction on Respect for Human Life in Its Origin and on the Dignity of Procreation* issued by the Vatican in March 1987. One finds in this document the most sustained indictment of AIH to date, and although I do not accept the Vatican's view that AIH is morally illicit, I do believe that the *Instruction* draws our attention to troubling aspects of assisted reproduction with which we must come to grips. Moreover, as surprising as it may seem, Vatican opposition to reproductive technology complements the resistance to assisted reproduction found in some feminist writings, particularly those associated with the Feminist International Network of Resistance to Reproductive and Genetic Engineering (FINRRAGE).

The Response of the Catholic Church

Although, ultimately, I want to focus on what the Vatican has to say about AIH, it is worth reviewing the *Instruction* in a general way first, for we will have occasion to return to this document. Moreover, it is nearly impossible to fully understand any particular section of this document in isolation from the whole.

The *Instruction* is divided into three parts plus an introduction and conclusion. The introduction sets out some of the basic presuppositions about human life and history that inform the Vatican perspective on human reproduction as well as some of the fundamental moral principles that will be applied in the remainder of the document in order to reach particular moral conclusions. The *Instruction* then goes on, in part I, to examine the use and treatment of human embryos given the technologies of IVF, embryo flushing and transfer, and prenatal diagnosis of genetic defects. Part II discusses particular reproductive interventions, such as IVF, AIH, DI, and surrogate motherhood. Finally, in part III, the Vatican takes up the relationship between the moral and civil law and calls for action on the part of political authorities to stop the spread of these technologies. The Vatican is uniformly negative about assisted reproduction. It condemns artificial insemination with either husband or donor sperm, *in vitro* fertilization of all sorts, surrogate motherhood, and almost all manipulations of human embryos.

The question that interests us, however, is not only *what* the Vatican condemns but *why* it condemns it. The answer can be seen if we examine the *Instruction* in greater detail. A close reading shows that the rejection of reproductive technology is supported by essentially two lines of argument, both articulated in the introduction in connection with what the Vatican calls "the fundamental principles of an anthropological and moral character."[5]

The anthropological principle set out in the introduction is that the human person is a union of body and soul. In the Vatican's view, a person is a "unified totality," and thus it is wrong to treat a person in a way that reduces that person either to mere body or mere spirit. It is particularly important to keep this principle in mind, the Vatican says, when addressing ethical issues in medicine because there is a tendency in medicine to treat the body as "a mere complex of tissues, organs and functions." Indeed, this is one of the central difficulties with reproductive medicine: it approaches human reproduction as if it were nothing more than the union of bodily parts, namely, of gametes.

The first line of argument is thus that reproductive technology is dehumanizing because it treats human reproduction as merely material. Since it reduces human procreation to the union of gametes, reproductive medicine is unconcerned with *how* this union is brought about. From the vantage point of medicine, noncoital procreation is different from coital procreation only in that it is a slightly more challenging form of reproduction. By contrast, for the Vatican, a conception that results from the union of gametes in the lab is a vastly poorer thing than a conception that results from a loving act of intercourse, an act that is quintessentially human in that it is at once physical and spiritual. By allowing for noncoital procreation, reproductive technology diminishes the full significance of human reproduction. It simultaneously turns our bodies into mere instruments of our wills—thereby dividing us against ourselves—and disembodies procreation in a way that sets the stage for the objectification and commodification of reproduction. I will return to this point below. In short, the first line of objection can be stated succinctly: insofar as assisted reproduction disembodies procreation, it is deeply flawed.

The second line of reasoning used to oppose interventions in the reproductive process is related to what the Vatican calls "the special nature of the transmission of human life in marriage." In the Vatican's view, since human procreation is the fruit of a "personal and conscious act," it is irreconcilably different from the transmission of other forms of life. It is intentional and purposive and therefore governed by laws. What laws? Laws, says the Vatican, given by God and "inscribed in the very being of man and woman."

As the language here suggests, the appeal is to a natural law conception of human nature, according to which we must understand the telos of human sexual life, marriage, and the family in order to discern the range of acceptable reproductive interventions. Moreover, the appeal is to a particular understanding of this telos, one in which intercourse, love, procreation, marriage, and the family belong together. In the Vatican's view, procreation is properly undertaken in the context of a loving monogamous marriage through an act of sexual intercourse. Here, then, we have a second standard by which to assess interventions in the reproductive process. Any type of assisted reproduction that conforms to the procreative norm just articulated, i.e., any procreative attempt that includes sexual intercourse between partners in a loving monogamous marriage, helps facilitate the natural process of procreation and is therefore acceptable. Any intervention that fails to conform to the norm is a departure from the natural law with respect to human sexuality and is therefore morally problematic.

If we now turn to consider what the Vatican says about artificial insemination with husband's sperm, we will see that the concern both about disembodiment and about violations of natural law are at work in the Church's opposition to AIH. The specific discussion of AIH is found in section II, B of the document and begins with a straightforward appeal to Church teaching on the nature of human sexuality. The first question that must be answered in considering the morality of homologous artificial procreation, we are told, concerns the nature of sexual intercourse: "What connection is required from the moral point of view between procreation and the conjugal act?" The answer is found in Church teaching on contraception. Quoting *Humanae Vitae*, issued by Pope Paul VI in 1968, the Vatican reaffirms Church teaching that there exists an "inseparable connection, willed by God and unable to be broken by man on his own initiative, between the two meanings of the conjugal act: the unitive meaning and the procreative meaning."[6] According to the Vatican, this principle of the inseparable connection, a principle "based upon the nature of marriage and the intimate connection of the goods of marriage," has implications not only for contraception but for assisted reproduction as well. It allows us to see that "it is never permitted to separate these different aspects to such a degree as positively to exclude either the procreative intention or the conjugal relation."[7] The implications for AIH are clear: Just as contraception separates what it is never permitted to separate by allowing for union without procreation, so does AIH make possible an impermissible separation by providing for procreation without union. The problem with contraception is that although intercourse and love may be held together, procreation is split away. The problem with artificial insemination with husband's sperm is that although procreation and love may be held together, intercourse is split away. Thus, the Vatican concludes, artificial insemination is morally illicit for the same reason that contraception is illicit. "Artificial insemination as a substitute for the conjugal act is prohibited by reason of the voluntarily achieved dissociation of the two meanings of the conjugal act."[8]

Although critics of the Vatican's natural law methodology have been quick to dismiss the Church's rejection of AIH as rooted in nothing more than an unacceptably rigid and indefensible moral framework, it is important to see that the Vatican opposition to AIH is also grounded in a second set of considerations. Immediately following the discussion of the relevance of *Humanae Vitae* that begins section II,B we return to the theme of the importance of human embodiment first sounded in the introduction of the *Instruction*. Not only is AIH wrong because it separates what it is never permitted to separate, it is also problematic because it reduces procreation to a mechanical manipulation of sperm and egg and thus neglects the embodied character of human love. In the words of the *Instruction*, "Spouses mutually express their personal love in the 'language of the body,' " and therefore, "in order to respect the language of their bodies . . .

the conjugal union must take place with respect for its openness to procreation."[9]

The appeal to keep procreation and intercourse together, therefore, is not simply rooted in a natural law reasoning but reflects a more general recognition that personal love is expressed in the language of the body and that an act of sexual intercourse that both expresses love and is aimed at procreation unites body and spirit in the bringing into existence of new life.[10] To create new life without sexual intercourse is thus to fail to accord human reproduction its full dignity.

Although it would be easy to dismiss this account of human reproduction as highly idealized and romanticized, it is important to observe that what stands behind this account is a very practical concern about the consequences of focusing, in Lisa Cahill's words, "so fixedly either on body or on spirit that the importance of the other is disproportionately diminished or seen in a wholly negative light."[11] The problem with noncoital procreation is that it encourages us to be so focused on our desire to have children, i.e., on our will to procreate, that we diminish the importance of our bodies in the reproductive process. The danger in approaching reproduction in such a dualistic fashion is that it ultimately reduces the person to the status of an object, thereby robbing an individual of the full respect he or she deserves as a person who is a union of body and spirit. In other words, because AIH separates procreation from intercourse, it bifurcates a person into body and spirit and treats the body either as an obstacle to be overcome or as a mere resource in the service of the spirit.

It is thus the very practical concern about the perceived consequences of the objectification both of the person involved in assisted reproduction and of the process of procreation itself that leads the Vatican to reject AIH. And those consequences, the Vatican believes, are quite clear: Persons will be treated as less than fully human; children will be thought of largely as commodities; and interventions into the reproductive process will be judged solely by criteria of "technical efficiency" in producing the desired product. The upshot will be the domination of technology over human reproduction, a situation in which persons will be reduced to objects of scientific technology.[12]

The Vatican opposition to artificial insemination with husband's sperm is twofold. On the one hand, because AIH typically separates procreation from sexual intercourse, it is contrary to the nature of human sexuality and thus a violation of natural law. On the other hand, because with AIH procreation is not a product of a loving act that is at once physical and spiritual, it reduces the human body to a mere instrument of the will and opens the door to the treatment of a person as a product. To our question, then, of why anyone would be opposed to a procedure that is apparently so simple and harmless, the Vatican has, in effect, responded that the procedure is not so harmless as it seems. Is the Vatican correct in this assessment?

AIH and Arguments from Natural Law

Let us take up this question by first considering the Vatican claim that AIH is a violation of natural law and therefore wrong. There are two tacks we could take in response to the Vatican at this point. One response, of course, would be to question the usefulness of a natural law framework altogether. Given the difficulty of identifying any concept of the "natural" in human sexuality that is not culturally determined, and given the impossibility of ever fully escaping the limitations of our historical situation, we might question the legitimacy of a methodology that allegedly provides us with moral absolutes. Such a response to the Vatican would involve an extended discussion of natural law theory and would take us far afield. Fortunately, there is a more immediate and less global objection to the Vatican position on AIH that does not demand a critique of natural law methodology itself but rather emerges precisely from a natural law perspective. Although this response to the Vatican objection to AIH will lead us to consider Catholic teaching on sexuality and parenthood in some detail, we should not lose sight of our ultimate goal, namely, to show that Vatican opposition to reproductive technology is instructive but flawed.

To begin to appreciate why a natural law objection to reproductive technology cannot be sustained, even on its own terms, it is important to note that the Vatican's position on AIH is so closely tied to its opposition to birth control that the two stand or fall together.[13] As we have seen, the opposition to AIH is rooted in the "inseparability thesis" that is at the heart of the Church's rejection of artificial contraception in *Humanae Vitae*. Moreover, as with its condemnation of birth control, opposition to AIH is rooted in a particular interpretation of the inseparability thesis, one in which it is not enough that love and procreation are held together. Instead, on the Vatican reading, the inseparable connection between union and procreation demands that every act of sexual intercourse be open to procreation and every occasion of procreation be the result of an act of sexual intercourse.

Those familiar with the debates about *Humanae Vitae* will recognize that what is at issue here is a particular conception of natural law. Once again the Church relies upon a narrowly physicalist, act-oriented natural law methodology to reach a particular conclusion. And just as the Church rejected the notion that contraception be viewed in relation to the totality of marriage rather than in relation to individual acts, so too does it reject AIH. It is not sufficient that love and procreation be held together in the totality of the marital relationship, either in connection to contraception or reproduction. On the contrary, as the Vatican makes clear in its discussion of homologous IVF, it is the morality of individual acts that governs. "The question is asked," the Vatican says:

> whether the totality of conjugal life in such situations is not sufficient to ensure the dignity proper to human procreation. It is acknowledged that *in vitro*

fertilization and embryo transfer certainly cannot supply for the absence of sexual relations and cannot be preferred to the specific acts of conjugal union, given the risks involved for the child and the difficulties of the procedure. But it is asked whether, when there is no other way of overcoming the sterility which is a source of suffering, homologous *in vitro* fertilization may not constitute an aid, if not a form of therapy, whereby its moral licitness could be admitted.[14]

The Vatican's answer is no. "Such fertilization," we read, "is neither in fact achieved nor positively willed as the expression and fruit of a specific act of the conjugal union" and is therefore "objectively deprived of its proper perfection."[15]

Clearly the Vatican is drawing on a conception of natural law that is focused on individual acts. But more than this, it is focused on the physical and biological structure of one sort of act, namely, sexual intercourse. Indeed, as a number of commentators have pointed out, the Vatican is so focused on the physical act of sexual intercourse that it appears to suggest that sexual intercourse is the only loving act in marriage. When the Vatican moves from the claim that a child "must be the fruit of his parents' love" to the conclusion that "he cannot be desired or conceived as the product of an intervention of medical or biological techniques," it appears to equate "parents' love" with sexual intercourse.[16]

Once we recognize how closely aligned the Vatican position on AIH is to the Church's opposition to artificial contraception—even down to its preoccupation with the physical integrity of sexual acts—we are in a position to see that virtually all of the arguments that have been pressed against *Humanae Vitae* are to an extent applicable to the Vatican condemnation of AIH. Certainly those arguments targeted on the biologism of *Humanae Vitae* are relevant. Yet we do not need an exhaustive review of the literature on *Humanae Vitae* to appreciate the problems with the ahistorical and biologistic character of the inseparability principle as it is found both in *Humanae Vitae* and in the *Instruction* on reproductive technology.

In fact, we need look no further than the majority report of the Catholic church's own commission on birth control, which in the 1960s studied the grounds for the traditional ban on contraceptives and recommended changing Church teaching. The majority report of the papal commission on birth control provides a powerful critique of the particular natural law approach adopted both in *Humanae Vitae* and in the *Instruction* on reproductive technology.[17] The document is particularly useful because it offers a persuasive rationale for change from within a perspective that basically affirms a natural law methodology. The fact that the Vatican chose to ignore the recommendations of its own commission does nothing to diminish the force of the argument for change made by this commission in respect of Church teaching on either contraception or, by extension, reproductive technology.

The majority report begins with an affirmation of traditional Church teaching on the importance of marriage and the family. It endorses the view that procreation is an integral part of marriage and that marital love and procreation are complementary in such a way that you should not have either one without the other. Indeed, precisely because marital love should issue in children, marriage brings with it a duty to be a responsible parent. And responsible parenthood may involve the regulation of conception in order to provide the "most favourable material, psychological, cultural and spiritual conditions" in which to raise and educate children.[18]

The report admits that this conclusion will initially appear to be at odds with traditional Church teaching on contraception, but a closer look, it suggests, shows otherwise. Because the Church has traditionally insisted that human sexuality is ordained to begetting and educating children, the good of the child must be a fundamental norm by which to assess issues in sexuality. It follows, says the majority, that "the morality of sexual acts between married people takes its meaning first of all and specifically from the ordering of their responsible, generous and prudent parenthood. *It does not then depend upon the direct fecundity of each and every particular act.*"[19] "The doctrine of marriage and its essential values remains the same and whole, but it is now applied differently out of a deeper understanding."[20]

That the regulation of conception is compatible with traditional teachings on marriage and sexuality can be seen in the fact that the Church does allow couples to avoid conception by monitoring a woman's menstrual cycle in order to avoid intercourse when she is fertile. A deeper understanding of church teaching on sexuality would provide for extending the means of regulating conception beyond those already allowed. Since responsible parenthood is one goal of human sexuality, the use of contraceptives would be acceptable when it served that goal.

Once we come to this realization, the majority believes, we will see that

> true opposition is not sought between some material conformity to the physiological processes of nature and some artificial intervention. For it is natural to man to exercise human control over what is given by physical nature. The opposition is really to be sought between one way of acting which is contraceptive and opposed to a prudent and generous fruitfulness and another way which is in an ordered relationship to responsible fruitfulness and which has a concern for education and all the essential, human and Christian values.[21]

In other words, the inseparability principle, as it is formulated in *Humanae Vitae* as well as in the Vatican *Instruction* on reproductive technology, is badly flawed because it focuses on the physiological integrity of the act of sexual intercourse at the expense of responsible parenthood. Yet if focusing exclusively on the act of sexual intercourse itself threatens responsible parenthood, then there can be no natural law justification for such a narrow focus or for the ban on artificial contraception that follows from it. Given that one goal of human sexuality is responsible parenthood, we cannot endorse a practice that frustrates the realization of that goal.

What would a natural law perspective that did not embrace a rigid inseparability principle require in respect of AIH? The answer can be seen in relation to the recommendations about artificial contraception made by the papal commission on birth control. Just as the commission endorsed birth control when it is used to promote the goals of marriage, especially those of responsibly begetting and educating children, so too would a natural law perspective support AIH as a means of responsibly pursuing parenthood. Just as the commission concluded that artificial contraception is not intrinsically evil and that the separation of union and procreation effected by contraception must be judged in relation to the totality of the marriage, so would a revised natural law perspective view masturbation and noncoital procreation. Masturbation would not be treated as intrinsically evil, and the absence of intercourse would be judged in relation to the totality of a marriage.

Moreover, drawing on the papal commission's reasoning, we might point out that to make a distinction, as the Vatican does, between procedures of AIH that facilitate intercourse and those that replace intercourse is like distinguishing "artificial" from "natural" contraception: such a distinction draws the line at the wrong place. Echoing the commission, we might say that the opposition is not between some "material conformity to the physiological processes of nature and some artificial intervention" but between reproductive interventions that promote responsible parenthood and those that fail to do so. One might even go on to condemn an interventionist mentality just as the commission rejected a contraceptive mentality. As with the prevention of birth, so with its promotion: interventions in the reproductive process should not be undertaken lightly or for trivial reasons.

My own view, then, is that an opposition to AIH that is rooted in natural law theory cannot be sustained. Even if we accept the usefulness of talk about the telos of human sexuality and marriage, and even if we understand the appropriate pursuit of this telos as central to human flourishing, it does not follow that artificial insemination with husband's sperm is contrary to the structure of marriage and sexuality and therefore an obstacle to human flourishing. On the contrary, a strong case can be made that AIH is demonstrably conducive to the flourishing that is arguably a natural part of human sexuality within marriage, namely, the procreation of children. And, as we have seen, the only time this would not be true is when someone construes the "nature of human sexuality in marriage" in a narrow, physicalist way.

Dualism, Disembodiment, and Catholic Opposition to AIH

If opposition to AIH on the basis of natural law considerations is misplaced, what of the Vatican's concerns about the disembodiment of procreation that results from AIH?

Here I think that the Vatican is on much firmer ground. Yet it is easy to discount the force of the argument from disembodiment for two reasons. First, the language in which the concerns about disembodiment are framed encourages an assimilation of this argument to what we have just examined in relation to natural law. When the Vatican says, for example, that in order to respect "the language of the bodies" spouses should not separate procreation from sexual intercourse, it is easy to mistake this for a natural law sort of claim because talk about "the language of the body" sounds remarkably like an appeal to natural law. And if the argument about disembodiment can be reduced to a natural law argument, there are good reasons, as we have seen, for discounting it. Second, when the Vatican talks about the domination that will occur if procreation is disembodied, it does so in a way that is quite abstract. Indeed, as I pointed out above, it is so abstract that it is easy to dismiss the Vatican's concerns as rooted in an excessively romanticized and idealized conception of marriage and sexuality.

Despite these difficulties, however, we should not dismiss the Vatican's concerns too quickly. The argument from disembodiment is not reducible to a natural law argument, nor is the concern about disembodiment based merely on a quixotic view of human sexuality. This is why I said before that in order to understand the Vatican's view about disembodiment fully we must focus on the practical consequences of separating intercourse and procreation and that one way to articulate the consequences is to talk about the objectification and the commodification of persons that results from this practice. But what precisely does it mean to say that separating intercourse from procreation will lead to objectification, commodification, and domination? To adequately assess the Vatican's concerns about AIH, we must answer these questions. Unfortunately, the Vatican does not provide a detailed analysis of what it believes the specific consequences will be if disembodied procreation is pursued unchecked.

We need then to supplement our consideration of the Vatican *Instruction* to fully appreciate the opposition to AIH that is rooted in concerns about disembodiment. We can get a sense of the specific worries behind the general talk of "domination" by comparing the Vatican's concerns at this point with those raised by a group of feminist opponents of reproductive technology who have also worried about the consequences of a disembodied procreation. Indeed, the general concerns raised by the Vatican are so strikingly similar to those found in the writings of some feminists that a comparison of the two should help us more fully to appreciate the Vatican's objection to AIH, even if ultimately Vatican objections and feminist reservations are not entirely compatible.

Dualism, Disembodiment, and Feminist Opposition to AIH

To get a sense of the response of this particular strand of feminist thought to reproductive technology, we can turn to a collection of essays that grew out of an international conference sponsored by FINRRAGE.[22] *Made to Order* provides a nice introduction to the concerns about the new reproductive technologies of those writers generally sympathetic to the goals of FINRRAGE. Its Prologue identifies three central questions that must be addressed by feminist opponents of these technologies. First, what is the future for women if the use of reproductive technology becomes widespread? Second, what is the relationship between reproductive technology and genetic engineering? Third, how is the impact of reproductive technology different for Third World women from those in the First World?

For our purposes, we can focus on the answers to the first two questions given by the contributors to *Made to Order*. What is the future envisioned for women if reproductive technology becomes widespread? One imagined future concerns a world in which the very meaning of motherhood has been called into doubt. It is a world in which reproductive interventions like oocyte donation and embryo flushing and transfer are so frequent that children may commonly have two, and perhaps three, mothers: a genetic mother, a gestational mother, and a social mother. In such a world it will make sense to ask who the real mother is, but there will be no obvious answer to this question. And, in the absence of a compelling answer, each woman's claim to the child will be tenuous. In other words, maternity may become as highly disputed as paternity ever was, and the upshot for women may be a significant degree of alienation from the process of procreation, combined with a real loss of power in relation to their children. In such a world, it is said, women will have merely instrumental value in the process of procreation.

What is worse, once reproduction is conceptualized as a "problem" to be solved by research engineers, not only is a woman's contribution to motherhood broken down into its constituent parts so that the various parts become more or less interchangeable, but women themselves get divided into parts. For the purposes of this technology, women do not have to be treated as whole; they have become valuable for their reproductive parts. According to FINRRAGE, this is precisely what has happened with the development of a commercial surrogate industry, and it is the danger that attends the establishment of egg donor programs. In either case women are selling their bodies or body parts as commodities. As Gena Corea has noted, the analogy to sexual prostitution is almost exact: "While sexual prostitutes sell vagina, rectum and mouth, reproductive-prostitutes

will sell other parts: wombs; ovaries; eggs."[23] Indeed, the idea of a reproductive brothel seems inescapable. If there are not yet houses of ill repute
where one can go to purchase embryos and women to gestate them, there
are brochures available containing pictures and biological information of
women willing to sell their services.

In other words, the development of modern reproductive medicine has
brought about the commodification of reproduction, and the specific upshot for women is that they are no longer treated as persons but as
products. And what is true of women is true of their children as well. The
logic here is clear enough. If women are paying for embryos or being paid
for eggs, the eggs and embryos cannot but be understood as products.
Because they are products, buyers will make demands on them. We will
expect our products to meet certain standards and, if they fail to meet these
standards, we will want to be compensated or to return the damaged
goods. In a society that sells embryos and eggs for profit, children will
inevitably be treated as property to be bought and sold. Just as inevitably,
it follows that different children will carry different price tags. As Barbara
Katz Rothman puts it, "Some will be rejects, not salable at any price: too
damaged, or the wrong colour, or too old, too long on the shelf."[24]

This concern about the commodification of procreation allows us to see
why the second question raised in *Made to Order* about the relationship
between reproductive technology and genetic engineering is thought to be
so pressing by feminists. If reproductive medicine promotes an environment in which procreation is assimilated to a manufacturing process and
the embryo is treated as a marketable product, the attraction of genetic
engineering will be evident. Genetic screening and therapy would be a sort
of quality control mechanism by which to ensure customer satisfaction,
and this increased pressure to engage in genetic manipulations will come
at a time when, because of greater access to sperm, eggs, and embryos
made possible by reproductive medicine, genetic experimentation can go
forward at a much faster rate.

We can see then why some feminists might be opposed to AIH. Since
AIH will allow for the genetic manipulation of sperm in the laboratory, it
facilitates the movement toward the commodification of reproduction. Yet
why suppose that increased information about the human genome and
increased access to human embryos and gametes will result in their genetic
manipulation? The answer, feminists say, is that there will be increasing
pressure to intervene at a time when the ability to do so will also increase.
We know, for example, that scientists have been working on the manipulation of animal embryos produced *in vitro* for some time, and clinical trials
for human gene therapy have already begun.[25] While these trials involve
only somatic gene therapy, there is little reason to suppose that, if successful, such therapy would not be pushed back to earlier stages of development. We know, for example, that the effects of odenosine deaminase
deficiency—the disease for which gene therapy is being tried—are mani-

fest in infancy.[26] The logic of therapeutic intervention would thus appear to demand that we undertake germ line gene therapy for such diseases if somatic gene therapy works.[27] Why wait until infancy to treat such problems if the appropriate genes could be injected into the fertilized egg to avoid the defect in the first place?

Moreover, intervention to treat the embryo would be consistent with a pattern of increased medical control over the processes of pregnancy and birth. "Human genetic engineering," Shelley Minden writes,

> fits in precisely with the medical establishment's increasing "technological takeover" of pregnancy and birth. During the 1960s and 1970s, medical doctors established control over nearly every possible aspect of the delivery of babies, including fetal monitoring, epidural anesthesia, and even the provision of out-of-the-womb life supports (neonatal intensive care) for increasingly premature infants. With the new technologies of conception, medical researchers are shifting their focus from the end of pregnancy to its beginning. The ability to diagnose and treat fertilized eggs would be a logical extension of this new research emphasis.[28]

That genetic manipulation of embryos and gametes would be consistent with other medical interventions in the process of reproduction is both evidence for the likelihood of genetic intervention and an indication of some of the consequences that women can expect if genetic intervention becomes commonplace.

The most worrisome consequence suggested by the authors of *Made to Order*, however, is the control gained by doctors over the lives of women if widespread gametic or embryo gene therapy is practiced. Women, it is said, have generally lost a degree of control when other technologies have been introduced. Why should gene therapy be any different? Electronic fetal monitors, for example, were originally introduced to treat women at "high risk" of obstetrical complications, but are now used routinely, often in cases where women probably do not need them and certainly would prefer not to use them. Caesarean sections were introduced to help (a limited subgroup of pregnant) women survive pregnancy who otherwise would not. They, too, are now used when they are neither needed nor wanted. This is the danger presented by the prospect of germ line gene therapy. Will a procedure introduced to test a relatively small number of individuals at high risk of transmitting a devastating genetic defect be expanded to include routine diagnosis and treatment of embryos? It is hard to see why the development and application of gene therapy should not be expected to follow the pattern seen with other technologies of birth. Acknowledgment of this point has led some feminists to wonder if the future doesn't hold the prospect of compulsory flushing and treatment of embryos before implantation. Would a "good mother" willingly risk a genetic disease for her child by refusing to test for and to treat genetic abnormalities?

This concern about the loss of control should gene therapy become reality points to the wider issue raised by the authors of *Made to Order*, not just about genetic manipulation but about reproductive technologies in general. When feminist opponents of these technologies imagine a future in which AIH and *in vitro* fertilization are widespread, where embryos are genetically tested and, if defective, treated, and where gestation takes place in artificial wombs, they do not see the utopian society envisioned by Shulamith Firestone in which the oppression of women has been eliminated because technology has overcome the biological basis of that oppression. They see instead a society that is more thoroughly oppressive for women than is our own.

According to this view, such a society would be oppressive precisely because it would strip women of this one traditional source of power, the power to procreate. Yet without other massive social reforms to accompany this change, the result would be a further concentration of male power and privilege. As Jalna Hanmer notes, this line of resistance to reproductive technologies may be surprising at first, but it is essential nonetheless.

> The defense of women's potential and real power in the reproductive process may seem to be a reactionary argument to some, particularly given the struggle in the early days of the women's liberation movement to remove 'natural' elements from our consciousness of 'What is a woman?' But we are not in a position to determine the direction of science or technology, nor do we control their empowerment through incorporation in the state. Therefore we must resist the use of science and technology to further shape women; our consciousness, our behaviour, and assumptions about who we are.[29]

If you want to see what the future will be like for women if these technologies become widespread, these writers say, look at how women today fare when these technologies are used. Although the justification for this use is that they "help" infertile women and that women request these treatments, the reality is that women's bodies are treated as objects to be manipulated, drugged, cut, and controlled. *In vitro* fertilization, for example, demands that women completely relinquish control of their menstrual cycles to doctors and passively endure the many invasive procedures required for a successful outcome to the process.

To summarize the feminist opposition then, we could say that the future feminists envision if reproductive technologies are pursued unchecked is one in which objectification, coercion, and loss of control will characterize women's lives. For this reason, feminists say, we must work to stop the spread of these technologies.

Although a comprehensive reading of *Made to Order* alongside the Vatican *Instruction* would reveal profound and irreducible differences between feminist opposition to reproductive technologies and that of the Church, the general claims of the two groups are substantially the same. As we have seen, both believe that disembodying procreation results in objectification, commodification, and domination. Yet whereas the Vatican *Instruction* remains almost genteelly abstract in warning against the dangers of disembodying procreation, feminist writers are characteristically direct and concrete about such matters and therefore help us to see the dangers more clearly. Where the *Instruction* is suggestive about the risk of treating our bodies as mere instruments of our wills, feminist writers are explicit about what treating our bodies as mere instruments means: it means that a sort of reproductive prostitution will emerge. It means that we will see the development of a mindset in which a woman's body is treated merely as "a field to be seeded, ploughed and ultimately harvested for the fruit of the womb."[30] Where the Vatican talks about avoiding reproductive interventions in which conditions of technical efficiency govern, feminists speak about what the reign of technical efficiency means: the possibility of compulsory embryo flushing for genetic screening.

So feminist objections to disembodying procreation help us to specify the practical concerns that lie behind the abstract denunciation of domination found in the Vatican *Instruction*. But now that we have before us the consequences that both the Vatican and FINRRAGE expect to follow from a disembodied procreation, what conclusions should we draw about AIH? Clearly the Vatican believes that AIH is morally wrong and ought to be opposed, and although they have not explicitly attacked AIH, many feminists apparently believe the same thing. But can AIH seriously be supposed to contribute to the process by which women are turned into reproductive prostitutes, children into products to be bought and sold, and men into brokers of women and children? Before answering this question it is important to see that by implicating AIH in this process, opponents of reproductive technology are not merely suggesting that AIH is the first step in what will eventually become a parade of horrors. The argument against AIH, in other words, is not considered to be a slippery slope argument that once we begin intervening in the process of procreation we will be unable to distinguish acceptable from unacceptable interventions and thus to control our own interventions.

On the contrary, what appears to unite Vatican and feminist opposition to all reproductive interventions is the belief that they are all dualistic and therefore seriously flawed.[31] Certainly the concern about dualism lies behind feminist opposition to reproductive technology, and whatever lingering gnostic elements may still be found in Church doctrine about human sexuality, it is a concern to oppose dualism that ultimately fuels the Vatican opposition to assisted reproduction. The problem with AIH is not that, while harmless enough in itself, it leads to serious abuses; rather, the objection is that it treats reproduction functionally and is itself dehumanizing. By separating procreation from intercourse, by dividing the person into intellect and body and putting the body at the service of the intellect, AIH, it is said, treats the person as an object; it treats humans as less than humans and is therefore intrinsically wrong.

Assessment of the Arguments against AIH

Is AIH dualistic and thus dehumanizing in the way opponents of this form of assisted reproduction say that it is? It is certainly true that AIH requires that an individual be prepared to treat his body at least somewhat instrumentally.[32] To provide semen to a lab in order to have technicians prepare it and doctors use it for insemination is surely to put one's own body and one's spouse partly at the service of the will to conceive. Surely, too, this form of assisted reproduction strips procreation of the intimacy that ideally characterizes the process when a fertile couple engages in intercourse with the intention of conceiving a child. At least this is how I experienced it. Indeed, perhaps the most difficult part of AIH for my wife and me was the struggle to maintain a degree of intimacy in the midst of a clinical environment that is designed to achieve results.

Yet does the lack of intimacy and the instrumental use of one's body of the sort we experienced make AIH a dehumanizing experience? I believe the answer is no. Although persons are indeed a union of body and spirit and although AIH can be divisive of that union, we often give priority to the spiritual dimension of the person, even at the expense of his or her material existence. We do this for good reason: it is the spiritual dimension of the person, those intellectual, affective, and volitional characteristics are most distinctive of the dignity of the human spirit.[33] Moreover, while AIH sacrifices intimacy in the process of procreation, it is intended to provide for the greater intimacy that can come from shared parenthood.[34]

Having said this, however, I do not want to dismiss the concern about dualism totally. Separating procreation from intercourse does have a price. The loss of intimacy in AIH is certainly one cost, though not one, I think, that is too high to pay given the goal one seeks. The greater sacrifice comes from treating reproduction functionally and, with this, from talk of "costs" used analogically to talk of "costs" used in a literal sense in which one must consider just how much money will be paid for the child one desires. That is precisely the danger when infertile couples and infertility specialists approach conception as a technical problem to be solved by technical means. When my wife and I abandoned the attempt to make AIH something it is not, we did so as pragmatists. Reproductive medicine does not encourage intimacy, nor does it make it easy. It is concerned, as it probably should be, with results. Participating in this world, we focused on results as well. We did not much enjoy the process of AI, to say the least, but we came to accept it on its own terms.

And therein lies a potentially serious problem. The terms in which reproductive medicine measures success are primarily two: the conception, gestation, and delivery of healthy babies and the profits to be had from the conception, gestation, and delivery of healthy babies. Both can be problematic. The problem that arises from making conception the overriding goal of reproductive medicine is that doing so easily leads to treating conception as the only criterion by which various reproductive interventions are assessed. In other words, once one has become goal oriented in the process of reproduction, choices about interventions tend to get framed exclusively in terms of the likelihood of the intervention successfully realizing the goal of producing a healthy child. And this is as true for AIH as for any other form of assisted reproduction.

This is why I said that the concern about dualism and disembodiment in respect to AIH is not intended as a slippery slope argument. Treating reproduction functionally is something AIH has in common with other, more controversial reproductive interventions. Once one has, so to speak, relinquished one's gametes to the doctors in order to achieve the goal of conception, it becomes difficult to judge various technological manipulations, whether sperm washing for artificial insemination or genetic screening for *in vitro* fertilization, or whatever, by criteria other than likelihood of success. This is precisely the problem: to treat procreation as the production of a product often results in the evaluation of the methods of production solely in terms of the resulting product.

This problem was brought home to me rather forcefully during the course of my treatment when I first learned about an experimental procedure being developed for use with certain forms of male infertility. In this procedure a single sperm is isolated in the lab and directly injected into an egg it would otherwise be unable to penetrate.[35] My initial reaction was one of tremendous excitement. Here was a treatment that could clearly overcome our problem. The fact that I did not produce great numbers of sperm or that the ones I produced were not likely to be capable of penetrating an egg did not matter. In theory, very few sperm are required, and the doctor does the work of penetration for them. The fact that such a technique involves placing an extraordinary amount of control in the hands of the doctor who selects the single sperm from among the many millions that even a man with a low sperm count is likely to produce did not even occur to me.[36] What is perhaps more troubling, however, is that when this was pointed out to me, I found no immediately compelling reason to object to this control. After all, I had been routinely providing sperm for a lab to manipulate in an effort to produce a collection that was capable of penetrating my wife's egg. Was selecting a single sperm that could accomplish the goal really so different? The fact that it is difficult to find a compelling justification for answering yes to this question from within the goal-oriented world of infertility treatment highlights one sort of problem that emerges when reproduction is turned into a type of production process.

There is, however, another set of difficulties that arises from accepting the second standard in terms of which reproductive interventions are generally evaluated within the world of reproductive medicine—that of financial gain. This remark is not intended as a cynical comment about the motives of infertility specialists but rather as a statement of fact about reproductive medicine. Infertility treatment in the United States is a big business.[37] According to OTA, $164 million is paid to almost 11,000 physicians every year for artificial inseminations alone. Add to this the variety of other infertility services provided every year to childless couples, and the total cost is at least $1 billion. There are some fairly obvious dangers that arise when decisions about reproductive interventions are made against this backdrop, even where decisions are not made exclusively on the basis of the bottom line. Given the magnitude of the sums involved, there will inevitably be competition for infertility patients, and with this competition will come a corresponding temptation not to present, fully and accurately, the chances of success with any particular form of assisted reproduction. Also, because the technology utilized in reproductive medicine is itself expensive, a subtle pressure may be exerted on couples to try interventions that are unlikely to be successful but that are necessary to amortizing the costs of the equipment required for infertility treatment.

This problem, of course, is not unique to reproductive medicine, and others have discussed the general dilemma raised here for modern medicine much more fully than I wish to do here. But there is another aspect of this problem that is perhaps unique to reproductive medicine, and it concerns the effects on the relations between infertile couples and their children when decisions about reproduction are so completely framed in terms of the costs to the parents of having a child and when these costs are likely to be enormous. Nancy (Ann) Davis, for example, has argued powerfully for the view that the use of reproductive technologies even to help infertile couples have their own children without recourse to surrogates or donors encourages an attitude on the part of parents toward their children that it would be better not to encourage.[38] Since I believe that Davis pinpoints a serious problem with assisted reproduction, I want to examine her argument in some detail.

Davis begins by noting that even apart from contemporary interventions in the reproductive process, attitudes toward children in the United States often unwittingly underwrite a situation in which the interests of parents are pitted against the interests of children. Because as a society we view the state as only minimally responsible for children's welfare—and welfare is defined simply in negative terms as avoidance of minimal harm—and because we expect parents to provide whatever above the minimum the child is to have, we create a situation in which prudent prospective parents must approach childbearing decisions at least partly in terms of a cost-benefit analysis. Certainly when the cost of children is understood to be a private and individualistic concern (i.e., not a concern of society), prudent prospective parents must ask whether they are in a position to bear the cost of having and caring for children. And in such a situation it will be reasonable for prospective parents to ask what benefits can be expected given the costs. As Davis puts it:

It is perhaps understandable that prospective parents should have such concerns in a society that assigns a very large portion of personal and financial responsibility for a child's welfare to the child's parents. But to ask such questions is to engage in a form of cost-benefit thinking in which the focus of prospective parents' deliberations seem to be on the costs and benefits that will accrue to *them.* There is thus a danger that the question of a prospective future child's well-being (or the lack thereof) will enter into the equation more as parental benefits (or costs) than as an important source of value (or disvalue) in its own right.[39]

The problem, in Davis's words, is that by thinking of childbearing and childrearing almost exclusively as a matter of choice and responsibility for individual couples, a child is turned into a "sort of private investment that a couple may or may not choose to make."[40] And the trouble with treating children as private investments is that "it encourages prospective parents to focus a great deal of attention on the question of a child's 'quality' even when that is not an index (or a reasonably clear indicator) of the child's well-being."[41]

If being excessively concerned about the "quality" of our children is a danger confronting anyone in our culture, says Davis, it is an especially worrisome problem for those who make use of reproductive techniques in order to have their children. Couples who have had children through techniques of assisted reproduction have generally done so at great expense, both financially and emotionally. It is not uncommon for such couples to have spent tens of thousands of dollars and years of their lives in the attempt to conceive a child. Frequently, this hoped-for child will have become the absolute center and focus of their lives, something for which they have made or are prepared to make enormous sacrifices. In such a situation, Davis correctly points out, we should not be surprised to see that parents' emotional investment in and expectations for their children have undergone a corresponding inflation. The costs have been enormous, and the expectations become so.

It should also not be surprising to observe how carefully attention is focused on the quality of children brought about through assisted reproduction. This is perhaps most obvious in the case of surrogate mother contracts where careful provision is made both about who is liable if something goes wrong and about what the surrogate mother must (exercise) or may not do (smoke or drink) in order to ensure that the child is not defective and meets parental standards. But pressure to protect one's investment is not absent from other forms of assisted reproduction. Minimally, this pressure may translate into a greater willingness to undergo amniocentesis and to abort "defective" fetuses if conception takes place. Given that couples may have exhausted their savings or already be in debt from their pursuit of parenthood, it is perhaps natural (and certainly understandable) that they would be reluctant to carry a fetus to term who will be a disabled child and thus an even further financial burden on the family.

More significantly, this pressure can easily translate into a greater willingness to manipulate gametes, either through genetic engineering or by other means, in order to obtain desired traits in one's offspring. Consider the prospect of such a manipulation in relation to AIH. It is possible to separate male-producing sperm (androgenic sperm) from female-producing sperm (gynogenic sperm) in such a fashion that one could reliably choose the sex of the child through AIH by inseminating with only one type of sperm.[42] If such a manipulation of sperm were to become an option for couples pursuing AIH, it is not hard to see how such couples might justify choosing the sex of their child as a sort of compensation for the ordeal of infertility and AIH treatment itself.

Further, we should not underestimate the way in which economic costs are likely to predominate in the sort of cost-benefit analysis forced upon infertile couples by the staggering costs of assisted reproduction. Although in theory such analysis should involve comparing all the costs and all the benefits, many of the costs and benefits are essentially incommensurable. Consider, for example, a couple struggling with male-factor infertility confronting a choice between *in vitro* fertilization using the husband's sperm and artificial insemination with donor sperm. The comparison of economic costs of these two procedures is relatively straightforward. Average cost of IVF per attempt is perhaps $7,000; average cost of DI is approximately $1,100. If, on average, it takes five cycles for either procedure to produce a pregnancy, the savings from choosing DI may approach $30,000. But how is one to weigh this concrete benefit against the abstract but perhaps real cost to the individual of not producing genetic offspring? Or, again, how does one compare $30,000 with, say, the sense of failure that many men would have if DI were pursued? The answer is that such comparisons are not easily made, and the upshot is that concrete economic costs are likely to take on disproportionate weight in relation to the nonquantifiable costs and benefits either to the parents or to the prospective children.

Moreover, even if one does attempt to find a way to compare the disparate factors at stake in decisions about reproductive interventions, economic considerations are likely to exert a subtle influence on how seriously one considers noneconomic considerations.

Consider once again the couple trying to decide between IVF with husband's sperm and artificial insemination with donor sperm. We have already seen that one consideration in favor of DI is the substantial savings that may follow from pursuing DI. But now suppose the couple is trying to weigh this benefit against the perceived cost to the child of not knowing who her biological father is. The couple may well be genuinely concerned about this potential cost. They may seek professional advice from child psychologists about the possible threat to the child's identity of being the product of DI. They may read about similar identity issues for adopted children, and so on. Yet, however seriously they estimate this potential future cost to be, it is being weighed against an actual and present cost. Perhaps ten or fifteen years hence a much loved daughter will be troubled by the knowledge that her father is not her "real" father, but if they choose DI they are almost certain to save between $10,000 and $30,000. In such a situation, it will be difficult to see clearly just how substantial the costs of DI might be, even if one is committed to taking such costs seriously.

Indeed, I can attest firsthand to the difficulty of this sort of comparison. As my wife and I attempted to weigh the various costs and benefits of adoption compared to donor insemination, we returned again and again to the fact that an international adoption might cost as much as $15,000 and take as long as two to three years, whereas DI would cost us very little—because most of the costs would be covered by insurance—and could move very quickly: two or three months to conceive and then the nine months of pregnancy. Further, because we hoped to have two or three children, the differences in cost and time of the two choices took on even greater significance. This is not to say that we ignored other costs in our deliberations or that we would have allowed economic considerations to override a concern for the future well-being of the child, if we had believed that a child would be seriously harmed by knowing that she was conceived through DI. Yet can we be certain that our belief that a child would not be seriously harmed by such knowledge was not subconsciously and subtly influenced by the fact that so believing might save us anywhere from $15,000 to $45,000? That we cannot easily answer yes to this question highlights part of the difficulty when choices about reproductive interventions are structured in the terms of modern reproductive medicine where economic costs figure prominently.

I noted at the outset of this chapter that there has been relatively little public controversy surrounding artificial insemination with husband's sperm. I hope this chapter has shown that, the arguments of the Vatican and certain feminists notwithstanding, there are good reasons for the general consensus supporting AIH. I have tried to show, for example, that the argument that AIH is wrong because it is unnatural and a violation of natural law cannot be sustained, even on its own terms. At the same time, however, I hope that the preceding discussion has also shown that, while not wrong, AIH is not nearly so unproblematic as many commentators on reproductive technology appear to suppose. When attention is shifted from the unnaturalness of AIH to the disembodiment that comes with the separation of procreation and intercourse in AIH, a number of problems raised by modern reproductive medicine come into view.

One of the problems, we have seen, is that to separate procreation from intercourse is to risk turning reproduction into a production process governed by norms of functional rationality. This means that the intimacy generally characteristic of human reproduction is sacrificed to the pragmatism of technical problem solving. More important, couples may begin to approach reproductive decisions in ways that are not necessarily salutary for either the couple themselves or their prospective children. The danger of commercializing reproduction and thereby turning women or children into commodities is real and worrisome.

Having said this, however, I hope it is clear that I do not accept the claim that separating procreation and intercourse is intrinsically dehumanizing. As I indicated, to undergo AIH is to act somewhat dualistically. Separating procreation and intercourse does indeed open the door to treating persons as objects and to putting profits before people. But to open the door is not necessarily to step through it. In other words, it seems to me that opposition to AIH is inevitably rooted in a slippery slope argument after all. If AIH is wrong, it is wrong not simply because it treats reproduction functionally but because treating reproduction functionally inevitably leads to treating persons as objects.

Yet my own view is that slippery slope arguments are not good arguments in general and that such an argument in this case is particularly implausible. The predicted "inevitable" slide from AIH to forms of assisted reproduction that almost everyone would agree are dehumanizing and degrading is neither inevitable nor even very likely. To accept AIH is not necessarily to accept IVF, DI, or surrogate motherhood, much less to accept reproductive manipulation that would deserve nearly universal condemnation. Nor is it to accept the commodification of reproduction. It is possible to distinguish among the various forms of assisted reproduction, and making distinctions and drawing boundaries is what moral decision making is all about. So while I note some of the dangers that confront interventions in the reproductive process, I affirm AIH as a morally appropriate response to infertility. We must turn now to consider other forms of assisted reproduction in our effort to further map the boundaries of acceptable collaborative reproduction.

2

Commodification and Coercion

The Simplest Case of IVF

I turn at this point from the relative calm of discussions of AIH to the din surrounding *in vitro* fertilization and the many reproductive interventions IVF has spawned. That there is unrest over IVF is clear. We saw, for example, that both the Catholic church and feminist groups are opposed to AIH. Yet for both groups the real target is IVF. The Vatican has talked about the "dynamic of violence and domination" associated with *in vitro* fertilization,[1] and Robyn Rowland's comment noted in the Introduction, that reproductive technologies turn women into living laboratories, was aimed directly at IVF programs. We can begin then with a question: Why is *in vitro* fertilization so much more controversial than artificial insemination?

Differences Between IVF and AIH

The answer to this question lies in the rather significant differences between what each of these procedures involves in itself and what each makes possible beyond the applications for which it was originally intended. *In vitro* fertilization is both more complicated than AIH as a procedure and more productive of applications beyond the procedure narrowly considered. While artificial insemination is a relatively simple process that gives rise to few variations, IVF is enormously complicated and generates many possible additional applications. Thus, with the advent of *in vitro* fertilization, we find ourselves in a position not only to fertilize a human egg in the lab but to freeze human eggs and embryos, to transfer embryos from one woman to another, to screen embryos for defects, and much more. This chapter and the next will be concerned with questions raised by *in vitro* fertilization and its myriad applications. Although perhaps the most serious objections to IVF technology arise in connection to its more extended applications, even the simplest case of IVF—one in which a woman's egg is fertilized by her husband's sperm and placed in her body—has given rise to many objections. I begin then with a consideration of the problems posed by even the simplest case of IVF. In the next chapter I take up offshoots of the original IVF procedure.

We can begin by noting the rather significant differences between AIH and IVF considered just in themselves. We have seen that the procedure for artificial insemination is remarkably simple. Semen is collected through masturbation, prepared in the lab, and deposited in the vagina or uterus by means of a catheter. Preparation of the semen may be complex, but the basic mechanics of the procedure are not. *In vitro* fertilization, by contrast, is as complicated as artificial insemination is simple. Although the specific IVF protocol will vary from clinic to clinic, a typical cycle will involve at least four stages.

During the first stage, a woman's ovaries will be stimulated with drugs to produce more than one egg during her cycle. Throughout this stage, the woman's hormone levels will be closely monitored through daily urine or blood tests and, as the time of ovulation nears, ultrasound scans will be used to gauge the maturity of the developing follicles from which the eggs will be taken. The second stage begins when the hormone levels and the ultrasound scans reveal that the eggs are sufficiently mature. At this point the eggs must be retrieved from the woman's body. This is typically done in one of two ways: through laparoscopy or through a technique dubbed TUDOR (Transvaginal Ultrasound Directed Oocyte Recovery). Laparoscopy is a surgical procedure requiring general anesthesia in which incisions are made in a woman's abdomen in order to introduce a variety of instruments, including a laparoscope, that allow for visualization and aspiration of ripened eggs from their follicles. With the TUDOR procedure a woman's bladder is emptied with a catheter and then filled with a saline solution. A needle for recovering the ripened eggs, guided by ultrasound, is then inserted through her vagina and bladder toward the ovarian follicles from which the eggs are again aspirated.

Once the eggs are retrieved, the third stage begins. This stage involves placing each of the mature eggs in culture with semen collected from the would-be father. If all goes well, the eggs will be fertilized anywhere from 12 to 23 hours later, and the resulting embryo, cultured for several more days, may then be ready for the final stage of *in vitro* fertilization, placement in the woman's body. If fertilization and cell division have taken place, and if the resulting embryos appear to be normal, as many as five embryos may be placed in the woman's uterus via a catheter. At this point the IVF procedure is complete and the woman is left to see whether any or all of the embryos implant in the uterine wall.

Even this brief sketch of the IVF procedure suggests one answer to our question of why IVF is so much more controversial than AIH, namely, its complexity. Complexity breeds controversy, for with this complexity comes increased risk both to the woman undergoing the procedure and to the child that one hopes will result. Consider the ways in which IVF poses problems absent in AIH. Of the four stages of IVF just described, only one part of one stage is shared with AIH—the laboratory preparation of semen—and most of the rest of the stages present potential threats to the health or well-being of the woman, her prospective children, or both. In stage one, for example, powerful drugs are given to stimulate ovulation, drugs that have known adverse effects, such as enlargement of the ovaries, and that may have adverse long-term effects on both the women and any resulting children.[2]

Egg retrieval poses risks as well, for both laparoscopy and TUDOR can be problematic. In both procedures infection is a potential danger, and with laparoscopy one confronts the additional dangers that come with general anesthesia. As we have seen, once retrieved, the eggs are placed in culture with semen in an environment designed to approximate the conditions under which fertilization normally takes place. Still, fertilization *in vitro* is not fertilization *in vivo*, and the possibility of damaging an embryo in ways that would manifest themselves only after the embryo had been gestated and brought to term is ever present. While it is true that so far there appears to be no increased risk to children born from *in vitro* fertilization, the oldest living IVF child, Louise Brown, is only a teenager. Thus, the long-term effects for women undergoing IVF procedures and for the children resulting from such procedures are still unknown.

Indeed, part of the controversy surrounding the development and use of IVF comes precisely from the fact that we do not know what the long-term effects will be. In the absence of such knowledge, many have argued that proceeding with IVF is a morally unacceptable form of experimentation on women and children. This theme was especially prominent in the early opposition to IVF, where, before the birth of Louise Brown, reflection on the potential dangers of IVF was entirely speculative. Paul Ramsey, for example, spoke for many when he objected to technological interventions in the reproductive process on the grounds that we could not know in advance what effects these interventions would have. "Prescinding from the 'good' ends in view," he wrote, "the decisive moral verdict must be that we cannot rightfully *get to know* how to do this without conducting unethical experiments upon the unborn who must be the 'mishaps.' "[3]

Admittedly, much of the force of this objection has been lost with the births of thousands of apparently healthy IVF children, but opponents insist that this procedure is still experimental and that we do not yet know the long-term effects of this reproductive intervention.[4] Anita Direcks, for example, has argued that there are direct parallels between the use of DES in a previous era to attempt to reduce miscarriages and the current use of IVF to circumvent infertility. Among the similarities, she notes an apparent willingness on the part of the doctors in both cases to assume that the intervention is safe until proven otherwise and that the birth of an undeformed child is evidence that the intervention is safe. Yet as we discovered in the 1970s, the daughters of women who had taken DES during their pregnancies in the 1940s and 1950s faced significantly increased risks of contracting vaginal and cervical cancer than women not exposed to DES *in utero*. So the fact that children appear healthy at birth does not mean that they have been unharmed by reproductive interventions prior to birth. Our experience with DES, Direcks concludes, should show us how mistaken our assumptions about, and how hasty our acceptance of, the safety of IVF have been.[5]

Moreover, while most of this sort of criticism has come from those concerned about the danger to children in IVF, others have pointed to the increased risk to women who undergo this procedure. For example, critics point to the fact that the early development and use of IVF in humans proceeded without prior studies of its effects in primates.[6] And while research and experimentation on human eggs and embryos were justified by appeal to the potential therapeutic benefit such research might have in treating infertility, volunteers were rarely informed that *their* chances of benefiting from the research were slim at best.[7] Nor, say critics, has the experimentation on women ceased. While it is true that the American Fertility Society and the American College of Obstetricians and Gynecologists no longer consider IVF to be an experimental procedure, nevertheless, experimentation goes on. As Patricia Spallone puts it,

> Women in present IVF programmes become the volunteers for various problem-solving experiments aimed at fine-tuning IVF procedures and increasing success rates, in the quest to know everything about the biological processes of women's reproduction. Many different kinds of fertility drug/hormone regimens are used in the various IVF clinics with no consideration of the long-term effects of such powerful interventions on women's health, and no questioning of the disruption of women's healthy life processes.[8]

Clearly then, part of the controversy surrounding IVF comes from the fact that many believe that IVF involves using women and children in ways that violate widely accepted guidelines about the need for informed consent in experimentation on humans. Whether this charge can be sustained is debatable, but it is not hard to see why the charge is made. Consider, for example, the following statement from the Nuremberg Code, the point of departure for most contemporary discussions of informed consent:

> The voluntary consent of the human subject is absolutely essential. This means that the person involved should have legal capacity to give consent; should be so situated as to be able to exercise free power of choice, without the intervention of any element of force, fraud, deceit, duress, overreaching, or other ulterior form of constraint or coercion; and should have sufficient knowledge and comprehension of the elements of the subject matter involved as to enable him to make an understanding and enlightened decision.[9]

In light of this statement, the alleged problem should be clear: embryos are unable to consent to the potentially harmful manipulations involved with

IVF, and women often agree to participate in IVF programs under circumstances that are arguably *not* free of fraud, deceit, or duress.

Objectification and Commodification of Women

As important as it is to come to terms with this objection to IVF, I defer
consideration of this matter until later. Consider instead an objection to
IVF that lies beneath the concern about informed consent and remains
even if this concern turns out to be misplaced. We can see the deeper issue
here by asking what the response of the critics to IVF would be if we were
to discover that IVF was in fact completely safe. The answer, I believe, is
that such critics would still be opposed to IVF and not simply because we
would have had to violate norms safeguarding informed consent in order
to arrive at this knowledge. Rather, the continued opposition would be
rooted in a conviction that IVF wrongs women and children, even if it does
not harm them. If I am right about this, one important source of opposition—even opposition couched in the language of informed consent—
is the belief that IVF leads us to treat women and children in morally
unacceptable ways.

   Here we join an issue raised in chapter 1. Recall that one of the concerns
raised in regard to AIH involved the potential for treating persons as
objects, and reproduction as a sort of manufacturing process, once procreation is separated from intercourse. In my view, much of the opposition to
IVF is founded on precisely this concern: IVF leads too easily to the
objectification of women and children. Certainly this is the concern of
those who oppose IVF because they believe that the embryo is fully human
and deserves protection from conception onward. To this group, the
willingness of most IVF clinics to discard "extra" embryos is clear evidence
that IVF dangerously objectifies persons. But this concern is not confined
simply to those who view the fetus as a person. It is also shared by
opponents of IVF who do not consider the embryo to be a person with
rights. Leon Kass, for example, has argued that although the blastocyst is
not a human being in a full sense, and certainly not a bearer of rights,
neither is it merely an object to do with as we choose. Yet, says Kass,
creating life in the laboratory leads us to treat the fetus in precisely this
way. Further, it leads us to look upon our bodies as mere instruments of
our wills. Unfortunately, Kass says, "this blind assertion of will against our
bodily nature . . . can only lead to self-degradation and dehumanization."[10]

   This theme is also found in the work of those writers who have opposed
IVF on the grounds that it is harmful to women. Indeed, as we saw in the
first chapter, one of the central objections of the FINRRAGE organization
to reproductive technology generally is that it reduces women to body
parts, thereby failing to treat women as (whole) persons. And if this is true
of reproductive technology generally, it is certainly true of IVF. Consider

just those manipulations I described above that are a routine part of IVF procedures. Women's bodies are monitored, drugged, cut, and confined. Moreover, women's bodies are objectified and reified in the process of treatment. Eggs are "harvested" as one might bring in a crop. Body parts are attributed a sort of individuality and intentionality; cervical mucus is said to be "hostile," the cervix itself to be "incompetent," and the list could go on.[11] Keep in mind as well that the invasive procedures of IVF will typically come only after a long series of medical manipulations of women's bodies. Many of these manipulations will have been painful, humiliating, or both. After hysterosalpingograms, endometrial biopsies, tubal insufflations, drug regimens, and surgeries—all done before IVF—it is little wonder that some women who have gone through IVF report feeling like a piece of meat.

The Dangers of Coercion

At this point we can summarize our discussion by highlighting the two principal objections. First, IVF is said to treat women as objects and children as products. Second, IVF is said to involve experimentation on women and children without their informed consent.

Although these objections are distinct from one another, they are also related. We can see the connection between them by considering the charge that IVF treatment reduces women to objects of manipulation. One response to this charge is to point out that IVF is no different from any other medical (or at least surgical) procedure in this regard. What critics of IVF point to, the drugging, cutting, monitoring, etc., of women's bodies, would be true of any modern surgical procedure. A woman in the hospital for an appendectomy would be equally drugged, cut, and monitored. And the reason these bodily manipulations are not morally offensive—either in the case of the appendectomy or in the case of IVF—is that they are potentially therapeutic and they are initiatives to which the patient has consented. Thus, in considering the charge of objectification, we are led back in a way to the problem of consent.

In large measure the debate at this point concerns the issue of choice. Supporters of IVF programs, for example, almost always defend such programs on the grounds that, however experimental, painful, or dangerous they may be, women choose to participate in them. Thus, it is said, IVF increases choice. By contrast, critics deny that IVF increases choice and claim instead that technologies like IVF are inescapably coercive.

Although opponents of IVF who claim that it is unavoidably coercive do not frame this objection as carefully as they should, I believe that we can distinguish at least three types of potential constraints on choice in connection to IVF. The first two have been vigorously pressed by critics of IVF, and the third has received very little attention. The first claim, to which I want to devote the most attention, is that, regardless of the information presented to prospective IVF patients, to make IVF available to infertile women in our culture is coercive. In other words, the offer of IVF is a *coercive offer*. The second claim is that, regardless of the fact that women are not presently forced to undergo IVF, growing use of IVF will inevitably result in forced IVF in the future. In other words, we can expect *coercive threats* to accompany IVF in the future. The third claim is that the existence of IVF structures choice in undesirable ways and thus leads to a coercion of unwanted choices, or what might be called *coercive choices*.

The claim that offering IVF to an infertile woman is a coercive offer hinges on the belief that choice can be coerced, even in the absence of force. This, say opponents of IVF, is precisely the situation when physicians offer IVF to infertile women as a form of treatment. Although there is an appearance of choice, it is merely a simulacrum. In a culture that so thoroughly defines a woman's identity in terms of motherhood, to offer a childless woman the "choice" of either pursuing IVF—even explaining the fairly remote chances that this will result in a child—or remaining childless is not to offer a genuine choice. Nor does the fact that many women agree to participate in IVF programs mean that they were genuinely free not to participate. Again, the fact that one was not forced does not mean that one was free.

In arguing for the idea of a coercive offer, opponents of IVF are simultaneously arguing against the traditional conception of freedom in liberal political theory. In other words, to believe in the possibility of a coercive offer is to reject the view that freedom consists in being left alone to carry out autonomously made decisions.[12] Affirming the possibility of a coercive offer is thus to draw attention to subtle forms of coercion and persuasion that are frequently obscured when the focus is on the principle of informed consent.[13] According to this view, the liberal understanding of freedom fails to account adequately for the way in which psychological or economic pressure may render the notion of choice largely meaningless, even when there is no physical coercion or threat of such involved.

Recognizing the possibility of such subtle forms of coercion, opponents of IVF have pointed to the fact that the reproductive choices of infertile women must be viewed in context. And the context in our culture is one in which a childless woman may perceive herself to be an unenviable social anomaly. To choose to be childless is still socially disapproved, and to be childless, in fact, is to be stigmatized as selfish and uncaring. In such a context, to discover that one is infertile can be a devastating experience and can lead to a desperate search to overcome this infertility at any cost. In such a situation, can we meaningfully speak of freely choosing to participate in an IVF program? If we cannot, to offer the hope of becoming a mother through IVF to a childless woman is a coercive offer.

Given the profound, if subtle, pressure for a woman to consent to an IVF procedure, critics suggest that to defend IVF programs on the grounds that they increase choice is ludicrous. It is especially so, they say, when one considers the fact that this technology is not generally available to single heterosexual women or to lesbians. Acknowledging this fact is tantamount to rejecting the picture painted by the medical profession of the benevolent infertility specialist working tirelessly to alleviate the suffering of infertile women by increasing the reproductive choices open to them. If this were the true picture, IVF would be available to any infertile woman who might benefit from it and doctors would be doing considerably more than they are to publicize and to prevent the various causes of infertility, including physician-induced sterility.

In addition to concerns about the potentially coercive pressures facing women in infertility treatment, critics of IVF have also pointed to the possibility of a more direct form of coercion that could arise in the future in connection with IVF. In speculating about the future, opponents mean to draw attention to the way in which past technological developments in reproductive medicine have often led to a loss of control for women. The use of ultrasound, amniocentesis, genetic testing and counseling, electronic fetal monitoring, and caesarean sections have all increased the medical community's control over the process of birth, frequently at the expense of pregnant women. Should we expect technological interventions in the process of conception to be any different from those of birth? If anything, a pattern suggests itself. What was originally introduced as a specialized treatment for a subclass of women quickly expanded to cover a far wider range of cases. What was originally an optional technology quickly becomes the norm.

Such interventions can be coercive not only in the weak sense that, once established as the norm, they become difficult to avoid but in the stricter sense that women may literally be forced to submit to them. We know, for example, that physicians have sought and received court orders to perform involuntary caesarean sections.[14] And at least one case has been reported in which a woman and her family were threatened with the loss of their health insurance unless she consented to amniocentesis. The concern in relation to IVF is that in providing access to human embryos, this procedure paves the way for widespread manipulation of embryonic material. For example, two laboratories in Britain have reported developing methods for screening IVF embryos for certain chromosomal abnormalities and for determining the sex of the embryo.[15] The concern is that as techniques for screening and treating embryos advance, IVF will become not simply a reproductive method of last resort for infertile couples but a common method of reproduction that ensures the production of a healthy child of the desired sex. If such techniques became sufficiently reliable, one can imagine an argument for compulsory court-ordered *in vitro* fertilization similar to that used to justify court-ordered caesarean sections.

I want shortly to consider whether the concerns we have just examined about possible forms of coercion in relation to *in vitro* fertilization should lead us to oppose this technology. Before turning to this question, it is worth drawing attention to a third possible form of coercion here, one that has received little mention in the literature on reproductive technology. Like the notion of a coercive offer, this form of alleged coercion is rooted in the fact that an offer of hope is made to an infertile woman or couple who have a powerful desire to have children. Like coercive offers, this form of coercion is "soft" in the sense that it involves neither physical force nor the threat of physical force. But unlike a coercive offer, where attention is focused on the potentially coercive social pressure that arises when motherhood is defined as the *sine qua non* for women, here attention is focused on the way reproductive technology itself structures choice. For some, the very existence of this technology gives rise to inescapable but unwanted choices.

Let me explain this problem by drawing on my own experience of infertility treatment. One aspect worth reporting is that while I did not feel coerced in either of the two senses previously discussed, I nevertheless felt coerced, *in some sense*, by the very existence of reproductive technology. That is, while I did not feel that my social identity was threatened by childlessness—and therefore that I had no choice about undergoing un-wanted treatment—and while there was certainly no threat, either actual or implied, concerning the possibility of declining treatment altogether, nevertheless I felt as if I had no choice but to pursue the reproductive technologies made available to me. Yet what sense, if any, can we give to the notion that, in being offered a choice, one loses options?

The very existence of *in vitro* fertilization changes the experience of infertility in ways that are not salutary. For most couples, infertility will be a problem they experience together. They want to have children together, and they have failed together. Yet infertility treatment distorts the reality of the relational character of the problem. Infertility treatment leads us to view infertility individually, with unfortunate consequences. The reason is that couples will often not be seen together in infertility treatment and, even when they are, they will receive individual work-ups and be pre-sented with individual treatment options. Now it might be said that pro-viding individuals with options increases agency rather than diminishing it. Yet with this agency comes a responsibility that may not itself be chosen and that reduces the prospects for genuine choice here. For once an individual is presented with a treatment option, *not* to pursue it is in effect to choose childlessness and to accept responsibility for it. From a situation in which infertility is a relational problem for which no one is to blame, it becomes an individual problem for which a woman or man who refuses treatment is to blame. Reproductive technology structures the alternatives such that a patient is "free" to pursue every available form of assisted reproduction or to choose to be childless.

I hope it is clear that such a choice may be decidedly unwanted. The problem, however, is that if the technology is available and it is offered as the only hope for overcoming infertility, such a choice is inescapable: one must choose. And a person may well believe that he or she has little choice. To reject *in vitro* fertilization, for example, is to accept responsibility for one's childlessness. Indeed, even where there is a supportive partner involved, the possibility for blame inevitably arises. Thus, a person confronting reproductive technology may well feel that he or she must at least try it, if only once. That was certainly my experience.

This problem is compounded by the fact that infertility specialists simply assume that patients will pursue all available treatments, and they typically present the variety of treatment options as just different points on the same therapeutic spectrum, distinguished primarily by degree of invasiveness. I indicated in the Introduction that this was my experience. Surgery, AIH, IVF, and DI were all presented to us as options without significant medical or moral distinctions made among these options. Further, as each option failed, it was assumed that we would move on to the next. In such a situation, to decline infertility treatment is doubly difficult. To stop treatment is not only to "choose" childlessness but to do so when the unquestioned social and medical expectation is that one will continue treatment.

The Force of Coercion

At this point we must ask whether the potential for coercion in connection with *in vitro* fertilization should lead us to oppose IVF on moral grounds. Does the danger of coercion, either in the present or in the future, preclude the moral use of *in vitro* fertilization by infertile individuals? The answer, I believe, is that the mere possibility of coercion should not lead us to oppose IVF *tout à fait*. Nevertheless, I also believe that the dangers of coercion are real, that some individuals are in fact coerced by the offer of infertility treatment, and that safeguards must be established at IVF clinics to minimize the possibility of coercion. In other words, we must balance the potential dangers of coercion against the potential benefits associated with IVF. Can such a balance be justified?

The answer to this question depends on how seriously we take the concerns about coercion. Although continual demonstrable coercion would be grounds for severely restricting access to IVF, there are good reasons for doubting that widespread coercion occurs in connection with IVF programs. Consider first the claims about coercive offers. The idea of a coercive offer is admittedly an important one. For example, it properly draws our attention to the fact that defining liberty in strictly negative terms, as freedom-from, is not wholly adequate. It also allows us a way of conceptualizing the sort of subtle, often economic pressure that may render an unforced decision also unfree. Acknowledging the existence of coercive offers allows us to say that "choices" made out of poverty or despair may not be truly free, however clearly the consequences of this action or its alternatives have been set out. It allows us to say, for example, that the woman who sells sexual services in order to feed her children may have been forced into doing so, despite the absence of interference from others.

Yet, while acknowledging the value of the idea of coercive offers in general, we must ask whether it has significant application in the particular case of individuals pursuing *in vitro* fertilization. In answering this question, the comparison to coercive offers in connection to prostitution is instructive. We have seen that Gena Corea suggests that current reproductive technology allows us to apply the model of the brothel to reproduction. Presumably she would also argue that reproductive prostitution may result from coercion in precisely the way that sexual prostitution does.

Let us take a closer look at this comparison. If we attend to the possibility of a coercive offer in connection to prostitution, we see that if we accept such a possibility we do so largely because we reject what Alison Jaggar describes as the liberal belief, "that individuals are fulfilled when they are doing what they have decided freely to do, however unpleasant, degrading or wrong this may appear to someone else."[16] In contrast to this "liberal" view, to accept the possibility that a woman who sells her body has been coerced by an offer of money for sex is to believe that the woman does not, and perhaps could not, flourish under such circumstances, regardless of what good may come of her actions. It is to believe that selling one's body in this way is degrading and that a person would not agree to be so degraded without some element of coercion. The notion of a coercive offer thus has plausibility here in direct proportion to the strength of our conviction that sexual prostitution cannot be a legitimate vocation desired by self-respecting persons.

Yet if we consider the claim that to offer IVF to a childless woman may also be coercive, we discover that for this claim to be plausible we require a conviction comparable to the belief that eliminating prostitution opposes no important human values. But this is precisely what we cannot affirm in the case of IVF, unless we simultaneously reject or devalue the importance of begetting and bearing children. Significantly, if we examine the work of those who have opposed IVF on the grounds that it may be coercive, we do in fact see a depreciation of the value of motherhood. For example, in an article entitled " 'Women Want It': In Vitro Fertilization and Women's Motivations for Participation," Christine Crowe argues that women participate in IVF programs largely because they accept the dominant ideology of motherhood in western culture, an ideology that includes the belief that biological motherhood is valuable. "IVF," Crowe writes, "relies upon women to perceive motherhood as desirable."[17] Or consider Robyn Rowland's explanation of the pressures facing infertile women. Under the heading "Pronatalism and the Experience of Infertility," Rowland writes:

> To understand the impact of infertility, we need to understand that we live within a society which says that it is good to have children. That is, one which has pronatalist values. . . . The exclamations of wonder whenever we see

something young, vulnerable, and cuddly such as a kitten are also reinforcing the desire for children.[18]

As I indicated above, I certainly do not wish to dismiss the very real pressures that confront infertile individuals in our culture. They are real and sometimes palpable. Still, it seems to me that both Crowe and Rowland—and many others who would follow them here—have confused the socially sanctioned belief that having children is valuable with a quite different proposition, namely, that women cannot be fulfilled unless they have children. To be sure, both these views are powerfully reinforced in our culture. Yet to conflate them is to fail to see that women may legitimately value children and choose to have them in full view of the consequences of this decision, even when the consequences include the bodily manipulations of IVF. In other words, even if women are socialized in our culture to define their identities in terms of motherhood, if we acknowledge the value of having children, we must also acknowledge that women may choose this good *independently of the oppressive ideology.*

To accept this point, however, is to concede that, regardless of the danger of coercion, we cannot oppose IVF altogether on the grounds that to make IVF available to a childless woman is a coercive offer. A woman may choose IVF not simply because she would feel unfulfilled if she failed to have children but because she values having children in itself. Admittedly, it will often be difficult to distinguish the latter case from the former, but unless we are prepared to rule out the possibility that a woman may legitimately value having children as a good in itself, it is hard to see on what basis we could justify eliminating access to IVF. Are those opposed to IVF because it may be coercive prepared to say of IVF what Simone de Beauvoir said of childrearing in one's home—that no woman should be allowed to have that choice because too many will take it? Surely, to agree with de Beauvoir here is to trade a "soft" coercion for a very hard one indeed.

What about the dangers of the other two sorts of coercion mentioned above? Are they sufficient to justify opposition to IVF? Certainly the possibility of coercive threats in the future should not stand in the way of an appropriate moral use of IVF in the present. The argument that the danger of future coercion should lead us to oppose IVF could take one of two forms, and neither is persuasive. First, it could be an argument to the effect that, in accepting IVF in general, we commit ourselves logically to accepting the future uses of IVF that could be unacceptably coercive. In this version of the argument, concern about future coercion is *not* concern about what the probable outcome of accepting IVF technology will be in the future. It is concern about what we have already committed ourselves to by accepting IVF now. In other words, in this version of the argument we should be concerned about the justification for using IVF today and we should ask whether the same justification could not equally well ground a coercive use of IVF technology in the future.

If we ask that question, however, I think we see that there is no good reason for supposing that current justification for IVF would in fact underwrite the sort of coercive use of IVF about which opponents are worried. Recall that one scenario envisioned here is that women will be required to undergo IVF as part of a mandatory genetic screening or therapy protocol, perhaps as part of a widespread effort to eliminate or to treat a devastating genetic disease. Whatever we may think of such a project, it does not seem to be justified by the reasons that have led us, if we accept IVF, to allow *in vitro* fertilization for infertile couples. While IVF does make the genetic manipulations of gametes and embryos possible, it is not for such manipulations that we allow it. Rather, if we accept IVF, it will generally be because we believe that begetting and bearing children is an important good, both to individuals and to society, and that physical dysfunction should not stand in the way of realizing this good, if we can avoid it.

Affirming the value of begetting and bearing children, however, is not the same as claiming that this value is overriding, that begetting and bearing children takes precedence over other social goods. Nor does affirming begetting and bearing children as valuable to both individuals and to society mean that it is equally or always valuable to individuals and to society. Individuals may sometimes value childbearing when society does not—think of contemporary China—and society may value childbearing where individuals do not—consider reluctant parents after a war. Acknowledging these facts, we are led to see that what may justify allowing IVF is not the same as what could justify requiring it. Thus, even if we accept the claim that eliminating genetic disease from the children we do bear is every bit as important as providing children to those who have chosen to bear children in the first place, we need not accept mandatory IVF to promote the former simply because we allow voluntary IVF to facilitate the latter. A much stronger argument is needed to justify mandatory IVF, and nothing in the argument for voluntary IVF commits one to making the stronger case.

The second version of the argument fares no better. In this version, opposition to IVF based on future dangers is a straightforward slippery slope argument. As with all slippery slope arguments, however, the case hinges on the plausibility of the assumption that we inevitably relinquish control the moment we step in a certain direction. In the case of IVF, the assumption is that accepting IVF, even in the most restricted of cases, will inevitably lead to widespread use of IVF technology in the future. From IVF to bypass blocked oviducts we will move to IVF to engineer custom-ordered children. Is this a plausible assumption?

Ultimately, I believe the answer is no. Yet there is an initial plausibility to this assumption, and it results from the fact that science often appears to have its own momentum. The sense of a technological imperative, that what can be done will be done, can lead us too quickly to suppose that we have no control over the technology we produce. But this is an illusion. As Leon Kass has reminded us, "Technological advance is *not* automatic. Someone is deciding on the basis of some notions of desirability, no matter how self-serving or altruistic."[19] And if someone is deciding, those decisions can be debated and opposed. Thus, the fact that IVF could be misused does not mean that it will be misused.

Consider once again the fear that IVF could lead to the development of genetic screening techniques for embryos that would result in widespread, or perhaps mandatory, use of IVF as a means of conception. To believe that accepting IVF for infertile couples in the present will lead to this unwelcome prospect in the future is to believe that the very existence of genetic tests inevitably results in widespread or mandatory screening. We know, however, that this is simply not the case. For example, although the technology for screening newborns for sickle-cell anemia has existed for many years, African-Americans have resisted widespread screening out of fear of discrimination on the basis of test results. Indeed, despite the fact that a panel of "experts" convened by the National Institutes of Health in 1987 recommended universal screening of all newborns for hemoglobinopathies, such screening is still far from routine.[20] Those groups most affected by the test believe that more harm than good will result from routine screening. Is there any reason to suppose that we may not reach the same conclusion about IVF in the future?

We have finally to consider the claim that IVF should be resisted because it imposes unwanted choices on individuals. I hope it was clear from our earlier discussion that, in one sense, this objection is a variation of the concern that providing IVF to infertile couples is to make a coercive offer. Again, the underlying concern is that IVF is offered in a context in which genuine choice appears to be limited. Here, however, attention is focused not on the social pressure to choose IVF but on the way in which the choice itself is now structured: either choose IVF and remain blameless if it does not work or accept responsibility for one's childlessness. I have already reported that I experienced the pressure of this choice powerfully during infertility treatment, and I have no doubt that others have been similarly pressured. Still, should the possibility of unwanted choices lead us to oppose IVF?

I do not think so, and I say this despite having been in some sense coerced by the existence of reproductive technology. Recall, however, the dialectic of which I spoke earlier. In suggesting that appeals to personal experience have a role to play in moral deliberation, I was careful to say that such appeals must themselves be subject to scrutiny. In this case, the feeling of coercion that may arise is being presented with an unwanted choice does not withstand critical examination. Consider the dynamic by which the choice comes to be seen as unwelcome and possibly coercive. The most salient feature of this process is that responsibility for one's childlessness appears to shift from "nature" or "fate" to the individual. Without reproductive technology, nothing could be done; one simply had to accept his or her fate. In other words, there was no choice involved. So the existence of reproductive technology does indeed create a choice where none previously existed. Nevertheless, it is a mistake to suppose that the existence of the choice shifts responsibility for childlessness.

Perhaps in some circumstances to unexpectedly and reluctantly have a choice does bring with it a degree of responsibility, if one chooses not to act. To find oneself at the scene of an accident at which one could easily rescue another with little danger to oneself will certainly place one under a burden of choosing to save. Yet even here the language of duties, rights, or blame may be inappropriate. In the case of choices about reproductive technology such language will be radically out of place. In this case we are not talking about saving lives, but possibly creating them, and certainly with *in vitro* fertilization we cannot do this easily or without risk. Indeed, even if we acknowledge the weight of a serious commitment of individuals to attempt to meet the needs of their partners, it does not seem to me that someone could reasonably be blamed for choosing not to undergo *in vitro* fertilization. Yet to restrict access to IVF in order to protect individuals from blame that is unreasonable would itself be unreasonable. We can certainly understand why an infertile woman who declines IVF may feel responsible for letting her partner down. Nevertheless, she cannot reasonably be blamed for her infertility, regardless of the existence of a possible treatment. It is thus the feeling that we should seek to overcome, not the technology. Once again, concern about coercion, while legitimate, is not sufficient to justify wholesale opposition to IVF.

Let me summarize my argument to this point. I have suggested that there are two principal objections to IVF considered in itself and that each of these objections has application to two distinct groups, women and children. One can oppose IVF on the grounds that it objectifies women and children, and one can oppose IVF on the grounds that it involves experimentation on women and children without their consent. Further, I have argued that concern about objectification is closely linked to issues of informed consent and that the three most persuasive ways in which it might be claimed that women do not freely consent to IVF fail to justify opposition to IVF in all cases. I want now to consider the challenge to IVF grounded in concern about the objectification and experimentation on children.

Objectification and Commodification of Children

We can begin with the charge of unjustified experimentation. In one sense, there is little disagreement here. Even those who support IVF must admit that the children who are conceived through this procedure cannot consent to it, nor can they consent to any of the risks entailed. This is one of the reasons that Paul Ramsey and others have opposed *in vitro* fertilization. We cannot be sure in advance that IVF will not harm the children created by this process. Hence Ramsey's conclusion: We can never know whether IVF is safe without conducting unethical experiments.[21]

One frequently cited response to Ramsey's concern has been to focus on the notion of harm on which it seems to depend and to suggest that the idea of harming a child through *in vitro* fertilization is more than a little problematic. The basic difficulty here can be seen in relation to a well-known example offered by the philosopher Derek Parfit. He asks us to imagine a case in which a woman temporarily suffers from a condition that would cause her to give birth to a handicapped child if she conceives while affected. Fortunately, if she waits three months, she will no longer be afflicted and will be able to conceive a perfectly healthy baby. The question Parfit poses is whether, if the woman fails to wait the three months before conceiving, she has harmed the handicapped child that results. The answer, he suggests, is no. It makes no sense to talk of harm in this case because, if the child's life is worth living, there is no intelligible sense in which he could regret his mother's decision.

This claim may at first appear to be puzzling, because we are inclined to say that, had his mother waited, the child would have been normal. But, as Parfit points out, had his mother waited, this particular child would not have been born. He calls this the "nonidentity problem" and argues that this problem arises simply from the fact that conceiving persons at different times affects the identities of persons.[22] So the reason we cannot say that the child in our example has been harmed is that we cannot compare his disabled state to one he might have enjoyed without his disability. Had he not been conceived when he was, *he* would not have existed at all. Thus, we can only compare his current state of existence to nonexistence. If he believes his life is worth living, we cannot say that he has been harmed.

The application of this argument to *in vitro* fertilization is relatively straightforward. If we cannot harm a person by bringing him into existence, then IVF cannot possibly violate a person's right not to be harmed against his will. John Robertson puts the point this way:

> At the time of the *in vitro* conception, there was no child with rights that could be violated. The parents have not caused a child who would otherwise be normal to be born defective, for there is no child to be harmed aside from the very act creating the risk of harm. The act creating the risk of injury also brings about the very being that is said to be injured. But for that act, the child would never have existed at all.[23]

In this view the problem with Ramsey's argument, and others like it, is that it relies on the problematic assumption that we can harm someone who does not exist. The conclusion that follows from this assumption is equally problematic. Preventing IVF does not protect the rights of the unborn because without IVF there are no one's rights to protect.

Although I do not find Ramsey's argument persuasive, neither do I think this response is satisfactory. The problem with this response is that it does not sit well with what I believe would be the considered moral judgments of most people about Parfit's example. Most of us, I believe, would want to say with Ramsey that the woman has harmed her child by not waiting the three months, even if, strictly speaking, the person who would have been born had she waited would not have been the same person as the person currently existing with a disability.

That denying the existence of harm is deeply counterintuitive can be seen by extending the logic of this example not simply to the standard case of IVF, as Robertson does, but to a situation in which gametes are manipulated *in vitro* precisely in order to create a person with genetic defects.[24] According to Robertson's reasoning, we could not sensibly say in such a case that the person responsible for manipulating the gametes bears any responsibility for harming the person who is created *in vitro*. For the act that brings about the injury is also the act that brings about the being who is said to be harmed. To quote Robertson again, "But for the act, the child would never have existed at all." Yet surely most of us would want to say that what the physician or scientist does in manipulating the gametes is gravely wrong and that it is so precisely because it harms the resulting person grievously. If I am right about this, then we are confronted with a situation in which we must either revise our moral intuitions about this case or revise our thinking about the concept of harm, or both. It seems to me that the preferable option is to revise our concept of harm.

Even if we do revise our concept of harm so that we can say that a person can be harmed through being conceived *in vitro*, however, it does not follow that Ramsey is correct that IVF involves unjustifiable experimentation on persons without their consent, at least not now. This last qualification is important, in my view, because the moral judgment I believe we should now make about IVF is different from what we would have been justified in making even ten years ago. The sad fact of the matter is that we did not know in advance what the risks were to children conceived *in vitro*, and we were very lucky indeed that the risks turned out to be minimal. Luck or no, however, the risks did (apparently) turn out to be minimal, and this is not morally insignificant. Indeed, it seems to me to take nearly all of the force out of Ramsey's objection to IVF. No conception is free from risk, and if the risk from IVF is comparable to, or at least not much greater than, the risk from conception *in vivo*, it will be difficult to sustain the charge that IVF involves exposing individuals to harm without consent unless we are also prepared to say this about conception generally. Further, as Leon Kass has pointed out, if one regards having children as passing on the gift of life to the next generation, one could justify taking some (minimal) risks on the child's behalf in order to bestow that gift.[25]

If wholesale opposition to IVF cannot be sustained either on the grounds that it involves experimentation on women and children without their consent or on the grounds that it degrades women by objectifying them, what of the claim that IVF should be opposed because it objectifies children, thereby turning persons into products and reproduction into a manufacturing process? I have already suggested that this may be the deepest concern of those who oppose IVF and that this concern may well remain even if IVF is demonstrated to be "safer" than conception *in vivo* and if women's decisions to undergo IVF are shown to be uncoerced. Is this concern sufficient to justify a rejection of IVF? The short answer here is no. If we restrict our view to what I have called the "simplest" case of IVF— within a marriage without freezing or destroying embryos—I do not see that IVF necessarily reduces reproduction to a manufacturing process or the child to a product. To bypass blocked oviducts by surgically removing eggs to be fertilized *in vitro* and returned to a woman's body is not necessarily to think of, nor to act toward, the resulting embryo, fetus, or child as a mere product. Nevertheless, as we saw in chapter 1, to technologize reproduction in this way creates pressure in the direction of commercialization, even if only because the costs involved may lead us to think about the children that result as economic investments. Thus, the short answer is not a complete answer. We need to consider not merely the simplest case of IVF but also those applications of IVF and IVF technology that go beyond the procedure narrowly considered. It is to this broader horizon and the expanded applications of IVF technology on that horizon that I next turn.

3

The Expanding Market

Moral and Legal Issues Raised by Extensions of IVF Technology

In evaluating opposition to IVF, we cannot stop with an assessment of the simplest case. Even if I am right that in many instances *in vitro* fertilization is now morally defensible, it does not follow that the use of IVF is always justified or that every extension of IVF technology must be accepted. We must take our cases as they come, and with IVF technology, they seem to come in ever more unusual forms. Consider just some of the developments made possible by the extension of basic IVF technology. Because IVF provides us with access to both human eggs and human embryos, we are now able to manipulate eggs and embryos in ways never before possible. We can freeze embryos for later use. We can transfer eggs or embryos from one woman to another, thereby separating genetic and gestational motherhood. We can screen for, and theoretically treat, genetically defective eggs or embryos. We can create embryos for research or therapeutic purposes. And these are developments that involve only eggs and embryos. Thus, even if we agree that there are no compelling reasons to oppose the simplest case of IVF, we have not ruled out opposition to IVF broadly considered.

Cryopreservation of Embryos

We must thus extend our discussion to encompass the broader context of IVF technology, and we can begin this task by considering one of the more dramatic innovations of the basic IVF procedure, namely, cryopreservation of human embryos. Although embryo freezing techniques are well developed in animals, their successful application to human embryos is a relatively recent phenomenon. The first U.S. birth from a thawed frozen embryo occurred in 1986, and the total number of such births worldwide is still relatively small. Nevertheless, we are likely to see a proliferation of embryo freezing in the near future for a number of reasons.[1] First, freezing embryos may eliminate the need to repeat egg retrieval procedures, thereby reducing the risk of IVF to women. Second, embryo freezing may reduce the chances of multiple pregnancies and their attendant risks because the pressure to place all fertilized eggs back into the woman's body is reduced. Third, embryo freezing may appear increasingly attractive as a sort of preventive measure to couples who are at greater risk of infertility due to workplace hazards, medical therapies (e.g., cancer radiation therapy), or simply delayed childbearing. So although embryo freezing has never been part of the standard IVF protocol, we can expect it shortly to become a routine adjunct of IVF practice.

Moreover, the ability to freeze embryos expands the horizons of reproductive possibilities. Embryo donation, or what some call embryo adoption, is more easily facilitated. So-called embryo banking, that is, the development of commercial cryopreservation centers where embryos can be purchased for immediate implantation or stored as insurance against future infertility, becomes a possibility. Embryo freezing also increases the likelihood for genetic screening of embryos, for the results of currently available tests are not obtainable until a point at which implantation cannot take place. Reliable freezing and thawing techniques would thus make screening a realistic possibility because embryos could be biopsied and then frozen until test results were back. In short, the development of human embryo freezing techniques is precisely the sort of extension of reproductive technology that IVF makes possible and that in turn makes IVF controversial.

If we consider this extension in light of the objections to IVF examined in the previous chapter, it is not hard to see why the advent of cryopreservation of human embryos might be opposed. Concerns about experimentation and objectification both appear to be legitimate in this context. A case could certainly be made, for example, that although embryo freezing may make IVF safer for women, its effects on the children who result are largely unknown. In the absence of reliable information about the dangers to children, cryopreservation could reasonably be said to involve unjustified experimentation on them. While this is a reasonable concern, it is not one on which I wish to focus. Instead, let's consider the novel issues raised by cryopreservation, namely, how to conceptualize the status of a frozen embryo and the nature of our control over it. Both questions lead directly back to concerns about objectification and commodification.

Two well-known cases highlight the unusual difficulties posed by freezing human embryos. The first involved a wealthy Los Angeles couple, Mario and Elsa Rios, who sought a child through IVF at the Victoria Medical Center in Melbourne, Australia. Unable to conceive on their own, the couple opted to pursue IVF with donor sperm. In 1981, three of Mrs. Rios's eggs were successfully fertilized. Two of these embryos were frozen, and the third was placed in Mrs. Rios's body but was not carried to term. Both Mr. and Mrs. Rios were later killed in a plane crash. The Melbourne center was faced with the question of what to do with the two remaining (frozen) embryos. This was complicated by the fact that the Rioses had not executed a will and had left no instructions about the disposition of the embryos. The case raised the questions of status and disposition in dramatic fashion. Were the embryos potential heirs to the Rios fortune? Were they property to be divided according to California laws of intestacy? Were they potential persons who ought to be given the chance to live? Were they merely human tissue to be disposed of at the convenience of the Victoria Center? What should be done with them?

The second case posed many of the same questions. Here the central actors were Mary Sue and Junior Davis, who turned to *in vitro* fertilization in 1985 after five tubal pregnancies and surgery that rendered Mrs. Davis incapable of natural conception. Mary Sue Davis underwent six cycles of IVF, all of them unsuccessful. The Davises then sought to adopt a child, but this, too, was unsuccessful. In the fall of 1988, the Davises decided to try *in vitro* fertilization once again, in part because cryopreservation had become an option. It would thus be possible to freeze embryos, for future attempts, if the initial cycle of IVF failed. In December 1988, nine ova from Mrs. Davis were inseminated *in vitro* with Mr. Davis's sperm and nine apparently healthy embryos developed. Two of these were placed in Mrs. Davis, and the remaining seven were frozen.

Unfortunately, the two embryos failed to develop, and before any of the frozen embryos could be transferred to Mrs. Davis's body, as planned, the Davises separated. Junior Davis then brought suit against Mary Sue Davis to block the transfer of frozen embryos. He asked the court to give Mrs. Davis and him joint custody of the embryos, to prohibit Mrs. Davis from having the embryos implanted without his consent, or, if they were to be implanted, to ensure that they only be implanted in Mrs. Davis's body. Once again questions of status and disposition were spotlighted. Were the embryos property, as Junior Davis claimed, or were they children, as Mary Sue Davis insisted? What role should the IVF center have in the disposition of the embryos? How should the frozen embryos be treated under the law?

One of the interesting facts about these two cases is that their outcomes were similar and presupposed similar solutions. In the Rios case, a California superior court declared Elsa Rios's mother to be the sole heir to the Rios fortune, and the Victoria Center subsequently announced that the embryos would be implanted when a suitable recipient was found. In the Davis case, a Tennessee judge ruled that the embryos were not property and awarded custody of the embryos to Mrs. Davis for implantation. Thus, the embryos were viewed as more than property and were given a chance to develop beyond their frozen state.

These outcomes, however, should not blind us to the fact that these questions were raised at all only because of developments in IVF technology. To be sure, IVF itself set the stage for such questions by providing the sort of access to embryos that makes concerns about testing, freezing, thawing, and altering embryos meaningful. Yet testing, freezing, thawing, and altering embryos were not part of the original IVF protocol, and we must ask how reproductive medicine has been affected by these developments and how it will be affected as these interventions become more and more routine.

The Davis Case and the Trend toward Commodification

If we attend just to the general direction in which developments in IVF technology appear to be carrying reproductive medicine, I think the answer is relatively clear: there is growing pressure (and opportunity) for control as well as movement toward the commodification of reproduction. Consider the Davis case once again. Although the trial judge ultimately held that the frozen embryos were not property but rather children whose best interests the court must take into account, he reached this finding in direct opposition to the testimony of three of the four expert witnesses in reproductive medicine. Moreover, it is particularly worth noting that all three of these witnesses drew upon a report of the Ethics Committee of the American Fertility Society (AFS) that endorsed both cryopreservation and a distinction between preembryos and embryos. Indeed, the question of whether the court should recognize the distinction between embryos and preembryos promulgated by the American Fertility Society became so crucial to the case that it is worth reviewing.

The issue arose in the Davis case because witnesses for the plaintiff, Mr. Davis, argued that the frozen embryos, although human, were not in existence. Rather, these witnesses suggested that the frozen embryos were at a stage of development where the most that could be said of them is that they had a potential for life. In pressing this claim, the witnesses invoked the distinction drawn by the American Fertility Society between pre-embryos and embryos. Briefly summarized, the AFS position is as follows. There is substantial biologic evidence that developmental singleness does not arise until at least the time of implantation of the embryo in the uterus and the development of the embryonic axis.[2] Prior to that point, cellular differentiation relates primarily to physiologic interaction with the mother, i.e., with the development of extra-embryonic structures, and not with the development of a single, distinct individual. For this reason, it makes sense to distinguish a preembryo from an embryo and to assign these stages a different moral and legal status. A preembryo is thus defined as "a product of gametic union from fertilization to the appearance of the embryonic axis,"[3] and an embryo is defined as "the rudiment of the whole being that first appears in the second week after fertilization and continues to develop."[4] Correspondingly, the AFS concludes that the preembryo, while more than mere human tissue, is not a person and thus may, within limits, be disposed of as the genetic providers see fit.[5]

Although the AFS was careful to say that it did not believe that distinguishing preembryos from embryos implied "a moral evaluation of the preembryo,"[6] and although it rejected the moral view of the preembryo as "no different from that of any other human tissue,"[7] there is no question but that Mr. Davis invoked this distinction to support his claim that the frozen embryos constituted property jointly owned by his wife and himself. And he was upheld in this by testimony from the legal scholar John Robertson, a member of the AFS Ethics Committee, which had formulated the AFS guidelines on frozen embryos. Although Robertson did not appear as an AFS spokesperson, he was, nevertheless, considered an expert witness, and he testified, in Judge Young's words, that at their stage of development preembryos "might properly be designated fungible property." That is, preembryos might properly be treated as interchangeable goods to which one has a right of possession and disposal.

As I already indicated, the judge did not accept this view of the fetus and explicitly ruled that AFS guidelines were not binding on the court, that the distinction between preembryos and embryos is a false one, that human life begins at conception, and that the common law doctrine of *pares patria* controls children, *in vitro*. Nevertheless, the judge could have ruled differently and would have so ruled had he listened to the testimony of those who most faithfully represented the mainstream view within reproductive medicine.[8] That is the significant point: there is a substantial and growing consensus that individuals have a right to reproduce noncoitally or collaboratively even when this involves treating embryos as quasi-property or contracting with third parties for contributions of gametes or gestational services.

Constitutional Considerations of Collaborative Reproduction

Consider, for example, the position of John Robertson, perhaps the most articulate and influential advocate for this view. Robertson served on the Ethics Committee of the American Fertility Society, whose guidelines we have already discussed, he was involved with the report of the Office of Technology Assessment on medical and social issues in infertility, and he has written prolifically and eloquently in defense of the view that noncoital reproduction is a basic constitutional right that cannot be restricted by the state without evidence of substantial harm flowing from such reproductive interventions. Indeed, his writings have been so influential, it is worth examining them at length.

It is important at the outset of this examination to be clear that although Robertson is a legal scholar and has carefully sought to clarify the legal status of noncoital and collaborative reproduction, he has also clearly intended to do much more than simply explicate the law. He has wanted to articulate and defend a particular view not only of the legal but of the moral status of assisted reproduction. Even a cursory review of his work makes this dual focus clear. We find articles with titles like "Technology and Motherhood: Legal and Ethical Issues in Human Egg Donation" and "Ethical and Legal Issues in Cryopreservation of Human Embryos." We find section headings such as "Normative Issues," "The Moral and Legal Status of Preimplantation Embryos," and "Reproductive Responsibility and Harm to Offspring." And the list could go on. We must begin then by distinguishing Robertson's views on the legal status of assisted reproduction from his views on its moral status. We will see, however, that he does not always distinguish these two as carefully as he should.

Robertson's views of what the legal status of assisted reproduction is and what it should be in the future have been developed in a series of essays written over the past ten to twelve years, in which he has systematically addressed most of the significant issues connected to collaborative reproduction. Although there is some variation in theme and emphasis among the essays, a fairly consistent picture emerges. In Robertson's view, collaborative procreation must be placed squarely in the context of reproductive rights generally. This means that in attempting to delineate the rights and responsibilities attaching to assisted reproduction, we must distinguish various aspects of procreative autonomy, three of which Robertson highlights. First, procreative autonomy involves the right not to procreate. Second, it involves the right to procreate. Third, it involves the right to control the characteristics of offspring who result from the exercise of the second right.[9]

In considering the legal status of noncoital reproduction we are concerned primarily with questions about the positive right to procreate and whether, if such a right exists, it protects the liberty to determine the genetic characteristics of offspring. Robertson argues that, given the paucity of actual court cases concerning the positive right *to* procreate, we must not neglect those cases that clearly establish the right *not to* procreate, for these two rights are related. As Robertson puts it, "This well-established right [not to procreate] implies the freedom not to exercise it and, hence, the freedom to procreate."[10] To be sure, there is some asymmetry between these rights because eliminating the negative right imposes burdens, whereas eliminating the positive right simply blocks access to benefits. Nevertheless, the two rights do appear to be logically connected. Thus, the fact that the Supreme Court has recognized the one suggests that it may well come explicitly to recognize the other.

There are other indications to this effect as well. Although there are no Supreme Court cases directly on point, the Court has, in *dicta*, repeatedly suggested that a right to procreate is constitutionally protected. In a number of Court cases we find language, in Robertson's words, "broad enough to encompass [a right to] coital, and most noncoital, forms of reproduction."[11] For example, cases like *Meyer v. Nebraska* and *Stanley v. Illinois* appear to support this conclusion. In some cases, the language is striking. In *Eisenstadt v. Baird*, for example, Justice Brennan is quite explicit:

"If the right of privacy means anything, it is the right of the individual, married or single, to be free of unwarranted governmental intrusion into matters so fundamentally affecting a person as the decision to bear or beget a child."[12]

So there is reason to believe that the Supreme Court would recognize a right to procreate, at least the right of a married couple to procreate through natural means. Yet, according to Robertson, if there is a right to procreate coitally, there is also reason to believe that a right to procreate noncoitally would be protected as well. As Robertson points out, the interests that would be protected by a right to coital reproduction are no less in evidence when procreation takes place noncoitally. In other words, the freedom to create and rear biological descendants is important to individuals and to society whether the conception of descendants takes place *in vivo* or *in vitro*, whether it is assisted by medical intervention or not.

Moreover, if we attend more precisely to the interests at stake here, we see that the importance of procreation to individuals may be derived from a number of sources. Although typically genetic, gestational, and social parenthood are combined to create a powerful procreative experience, each may have value to individuals independently of the others.[13] Some people may find satisfaction in simply passing on genes to biological offspring, thereby establishing a connection to future generations. Others may value the experience of gestating a child, without a need for genetic connection or the rewards of rearing a child. Still others may value the experience of rearing a child without concern for genetic or gestational connection. Thus Robertson concludes that full procreative freedom would include "the right to separate the genetic, gestational, or social components of reproduction and to recombine them in collaboration with others."[14] Or, in more straightforward language, full procreative autonomy would include the freedom "to reproduce when, with whom, and by what means one chooses."[15]

Taken in its strongest form this claim suggests that individuals have rights both to create biological descendants without rearing them and to gestate children without rearing them, and both suggestions seem problematic. A more modest reading of Robertson's claim is that a very strong case can be made for the right to procreate noncoitally when genetic, gestational, and social parenthood are held together and that, while not as strong, a good case can be made for a right to procreate collaboratively when genetic, gestational, and social parenthood cannot be held together. In this reading, the right to procreate would not necessarily protect the liberty to become a genetic or gestational parent apart from the responsibilities associated with rearing children, but it would, as Robertson says at one point, protect the freedom to "acquire a child for rearing purposes," by any "medical or social means necessary to do so."[16]

Establishing a case for the right to procreate, however, is only part of a complete legal analysis of assisted reproduction. It must be accompanied by a discussion of what restrictions, if any, the state may place on the exercise of this right. Much of Robertson's work on the legal status of the right to procreate is taken up with this task of identifying possible restrictions. According to Robertson, the basic legal issue is quite clear. If a right to procreate is constitutionally protected, a compelling state interest will need to be demonstrated in order to justify a restriction on the exercise of that right. The crucial question is whether a compelling state interest in restricting noncoital or collaborative reproduction can be demonstrated. Robertson identifies a handful of candidates, but rejects them all. States may have an interest in (1) safeguarding embryos, (2) protecting offspring from physical or psychosocial harm, (3) protecting collaborators from physical or psychosocial harm, (4) preserving the family, or (5) avoiding the reification of reproduction. Let us consider each of these in turn.

Safeguarding Embryos

Even if a right to procreate is constitutionally protected, the state may have an interest in protecting the embryos that are created, observed, tested, manipulated, etc., in the process of noncoital reproduction. We have already seen one expression of this view in the Davis case. In ruling for Mary Sue Davis, Judge Young held that the court must act in the best interests of the seven frozen embryos. Nor is Judge Young alone in this view. At least fifteen states mention preimplantation embryos in statutes regulating fetal research, and Louisiana has granted IVF embryos the status of "juridical persons" and forbids their destruction if they appear to be capable of normal development.[17] So a case can be made for regulating or restricting noncoital reproduction in order to safeguard embryos.

If we examine this case closely, Robertson argues, we see that regulation is justified either by assigning embryos the status of a rights-bearing entity, as Louisiana does, or by according special respect to embryos as symbolic of our commitment to human life generally. Neither position, says Robertson, is strong enough to seriously restrict the right to procreate. To treat the embryo as a rights-bearing entity is to adopt the view that the embryo is a person from conception and must be accorded the rights of a person. Yet in no other context does the law regard the fetus as a person, nor does the biology of early-embryo development argue for the extension of such rights in this case. The preimplantation embryo does not have differentiated organs; it does not have a brain or central nervous system, so it does not feel pain. At best, the preimplantation embryo has the legal status of potential person. Yet, according to Robertson, to appeal to the symbolic importance of embryos as potential persons as a warrant for state intervention does not appear to support any significant restrictions on procreative liberty. While protection from symbolic harm might pass a rational basis test for state action, it does not meet the more rigorous compelling state interest standard necessary to override the fundamental right to procreate.

Protecting Offspring and Collaborators

While embryos and fetuses may not be entities whose rights are constitutionally protected by the state, the collaborators in, and offspring of,
the new reproductive technology are. The argument is thus made that
states should regulate or even prohibit noncoital and collaborative
reproduction in order to protect collaborators and prospective children
from harm. Consider the need to protect collaborators. In theory, third
parties could be harmed both physically and psychologically. For example,
the procedures involved with egg donation or with embryo donation after
uterine lavage pose potential health risks to the donor. Potential complications include reaction to anesthesia, infection, and increased likelihood of ectopic pregnancy. Moreover, collaborators who contribute gametes but relinquish rearing rights may come to be haunted by the fact that
they have biological children whom they have never met. Collaborators
could thus be harmed physically and emotionally.

A similar argument can be made in relation to the children who result
from noncoital and collaborative reproduction. Although IVF is apparently
safe, the same cannot be said for the extensions of IVF technology which
we are considering in this chapter. It is simply too early to know whether
freezing and thawing embryos, for example, has any long-term negative
effects on the children so produced, but it may. Apart from this uncertainty, however, we do know that a risk of infectious or genetic disease
exists with collaborative reproduction. So, clearly, the potential for physical harm exists. Many have argued that the potential for psychological
harm exists as well. The possibility for posthumous conception or implantation—both made possible by cryopreservation techniques—or for
using donor gametes, embryos, or surrogates has raised concerns about
the psychological well-being of the children who result. Will confusion
about lineage and genetic identity result in children who are not as happy
and well-adjusted? If so, it is said, the state may be justified in constraining
procreative freedom.

Robertson's response to the worries expressed about the potential for
harm, both to the offspring and to collaborators, has been to suggest that
these concerns, while important, are overblown. In practical terms, this
means that the risk of harm may justify some minimal state intervention in
regulating noncoital and collaborative reproduction but that the risk of
harm will not justify state prohibitions of assisted reproduction. For example, in Robertson's view, a state could institute a licensing requirement
for IVF programs in order to protect the health and safety of, say, egg
donors to that program, but it could not prohibit the program altogether.[18]
In Robertson's words, there are limits to "the state's interest in saving
mature adults from the folly of their own choices,"[19] even where this folly
leads to the risk of physical and psychological harm in collaborators.

Such reasoning would not, of course, apply to state interventions to protect offspring, but Robertson takes much the same view of this sort of intervention as he does about interventions to safeguard "mature adults": some regulation may be "proper and desirable," but a total ban is not defensible.[20] Despite the differences in circumstances, the conclusions are the same because, in reflecting on protecting offspring, one must distinguish avoidable from unavoidable harm. In many cases, if harm does come to the offspring as the result of assisted reproduction, it is harm that could not have been avoided. Hence it is harm from which the state cannot offer protection. Robertson's position here is precisely that which we saw articulated in connection to the "nonidentity" problem in chapter 2. If the only possible means of conception is through noncoitcal or collaborative reproduction, no harm can come to the child through assisted reproduction. There is thus nothing from which the state can protect the child. In Robertson's words, "avoiding the damage means avoiding the birth of the child."[21]

Preserving the Family

While concern about the deleterious effects assisted reproduction may have on embryos, offspring, and collaborators is probably the most frequently cited reason for advocating state regulation of the new reproductive technologies, it is not the only reason. We also find anxiety about alleged dangers to social institutions, and no potential threat generates more apprehension than that to the traditional notion of the family. Leon Kass, for example, has suggested that biological kinship lies at the heart of the social order and that assisted reproduction threatens the social order by threatening biological kinship. Kass writes:

> Our society is dangerously close to losing its grip on the meaning of some fundamental aspects of human existence. . . . Here, in noticing our growing casualness about marriage, legitimacy, kinship, and lineage, we discover how our individualistic and willful projects lead us to ignore the truths defended by the equally widespread prohibition of incest. . . . These time-honored restraints implicitly teach that clarity about who your parents are, clarity in the lines of generation, clarity about who is whose, are the indispensable foundations of a sound family life, itself the sound foundation of civilized community.[22]

Kass does not conclude from this perceived threat to the family that states should outlaw assisted reproduction. Even to proscribe practices like IVF, he says, would be "foolish." But certainly states should not foster or support assisted reproduction, either.

Robertson's response to this concern is to point out, on the one hand, that noncoital reproduction often reinforces the traditional family by enabling married couples to conceive and rear their own children and, on the other hand, that even forms of collaborative reproduction that appear most threatening to the integrity of the traditional family unit are not really very different from parent-child arrangements commonly accepted in adoptive and blended families. In fact, it is the power of the traditional image of the family, itself reinforced by reproductive technology, that fuels assisted reproduction. If anything, AIH and homologous IVF support the institutions of the family. Even where couples make use of DI and heterologous IVF, or surrogate motherhood, where third party collaborators are involved, the motivation is often to stay as close to the traditional family model as possible by ensuring that at least one of the partners is genetically related to the offspring of the marriage. Moreover, Robertson adds, even if a causal connection could be demonstrated between the coital and collaborative reproduction and the decline of the traditional family, this would not be sufficient in itself to justify state prohibition of assisted reproduction. One would also need to show tangible harm to individuals resulting from nontraditional family structures. If tangible harm to individuals could be demonstrated, state intervention might be justified regardless of the impact of assisted reproduction on the family. Concern about preserving the family is thus something of a red herring.

Avoiding Reification

A final interest that some have thought sufficiently compelling to justify state regulation of assisted reproduction concerns the consequences of reifying reproduction. We explored the basic concern over reification in the first two chapters, but it can be briefly summarized here as follows. One problem with noncoital and collaborative reproduction methods is that they technologize the process of procreation and, in so doing, dehumanize and degrade both the process and the persons involved in the process. A technological conception thus "demeans human dignity" and may well lead to the outright exploitation of women and children as procreation is turned into a manufacturing process ruled by the market. Unfortunately, when market forces take over, persons are reduced to objects whose value is measured largely in economic terms. Children conceived in this context are likely to be treated as economic investments, with the consequence that pressure will mount to intervene genetically to produce perfect babies. To reify reproduction is thus to head down the road toward a Huxleyan *Brave New World* in which babies with predetermined characteristics are decanted from bottles, a prospect that states have every reason to resist.

The problem with opposing assisted reproduction on these grounds, Robertson believes, is that it exaggerates the objectification entailed by the new reproductive technologies in order to make them appear especially ominous. But the fact of the matter is that "the attitude toward body and reproduction decried here is no different than that which underlays standard infertility treatment, indeed, obstetrics and medical science generally."[23] To be sure, IVF and its various extensions represent a particularly striking manipulation of the natural order to serve human ends, but we should not be prepared to endorse State regulation or prohibition of assisted reproduction unless we are willing to sanction State control of infertility treatment or natural conception, for that matter. For natural conception can also be a coldly calculated affair, as anyone who has tried to conceive by charting temperatures and menstrual cycles can attest.

Nor, says Robertson, is it fair to single out infertile couples who resort to technological help in conceiving as "selfish consumers" who view their children as valuable commodities. The costs of assisted reproduction are indeed high, both economically and emotionally, but this does not mean that infertile couples will come to see their children as particularly expensive luxury items—quite likely, the reverse. Such parents will see their children as priceless gifts and themselves as seekers of miracles, not mercenaries. Nor does it follow that, because reproductive technology creates the possibility of egg and embryo donation or facilitates surrogacy, it leads to the exploitation of women as mother machines. By contrast, Robertson points out, noncoital reproduction expands women's choices over when and how to reproduce and can thus be a source of liberation rather than oppression. In short, those who fear the nightmare of a brave new world and expect such a world shortly to be ushered in by developments in reproductive technology do indeed fear a nightmare, that is, a dream.

So a review of Robertson's analysis of the legal status of assisted reproduction reveals the following framework. On the one hand, there exists a basic constitutional right to procreate, whether coitally or noncoitally/collaboratively. On the other hand, states have an interest in protecting individuals from the harms that may result from noncoital or collaborative reproduction. The basic legal question is thus largely utilitarian: Do the individual and social costs of assisted reproduction outweigh the individual or social benefits that come from allowing assisted reproduction? When Robertson addresses this question, his answer is clear. The benefits of full reproductive autonomy far outweigh the costs of allowing such liberty. Indeed, as we have seen in our discussions of the potential harms that arguably constitute grounds for state intervention, Robertson believes that the dangers are more apparent than real. In fact, he often calls the objections to assisted reproduction "symbolic" in order to distinguish "purely moralistic and nonobjective" burdens from real and tangible harms.[24] The main impact of assisted reproduction, he writes, "may be on moral and religious notions about sexuality, reproduction, family, female roles, and similar value-laden concerns." Such concerns may be terribly important to certain groups in society, but when weighed against the benefits of ensuring full procreative liberty, they are "insufficient to justify infringing the fundamental rights of persons with different views."[25]

This sort of calculus leads Robertson to advocate a very full range of procreative liberties indeed. Not only should access to basic forms of assisted reproduction like AIH and homologous IVF be guaranteed, but so, too, should access to most extensions of these basic interventions. In Robertson's view procreative autonomy should involve the freedom to contract to pay or be paid for gametes, embryos, or gestational services. It should include the freedom to collaborate with others to divide the genetic, gestational, and remaining aspects of parenthood and to recombine them in novel ways of reproducing. Moreover, the right to procreate should protect the freedom to control the use and disposition of reproductive resources. It should protect the freedom to freeze and to store gametes and embryos, to dispose of gametes and embryos as one chooses, to create embryos for research purposes, or to provide fetal tissue for transplant. It should protect the freedom, wherever possible, to select the characteristics of offspring produced through assisted reproduction. In short, for Robertson, procreative liberty really does involve the freedom to reproduce when, where, with whom, and by whatever means one chooses.

The Conflation of Legal and Moral Arguments

Robertson's analysis of the legal status of assisted reproduction is instructive for a number of reasons. First, it helps us to see the logic by which basic interventions in the reproductive process can lead to more and more radical interventions. Indeed, we have seen that for Robertson the justification for AIH is the same as that for IVF with donor eggs, cryopreservation of embryos, surrogate motherhood, or virtually any other reproductive intervention. What justifies assisted reproduction when it is undertaken not for profit also grounds it when it is fueled by the prospect of financial gain. The same reasoning covers all reproductive interventions. If an individual has a right to procreate, then state intervention in regulating assisted reproduction should be minimal, unless the exercise of this right threatens the rights of another in some substantial way. But since embryos, at least preimplantation embryos, are not rights-bearing entities, the interests most likely to be threatened are those of the participants in noncoital and collaborative reproduction, and they have consented to participate. The fact that outsiders find noncoital or collaborative reproduction offensive or morally objectionable is not sufficient to justify state intervention. This is true whether we are considering AIH or posthumous transfer of frozen embryos or any other intervention in the reproductive process. In every case we must undertake a cost-benefit analysis.

Robertson's appeal to the language of rights should not mislead us at this point, for Robertson appears to understand talk about legal rights as a sort of shorthand for substantial interests. To assign a right to procreate to individuals is to adopt a presumption that significant benefit accrues from the exercise of that right and, consequently, that only significant costs will justify overriding this right. A right is thus a sort of multiplier in the utilitarian calculus by which the legal status of assisted reproduction is adjudicated. In other words, attribution of a right to procreate noncoitally or collaboratively *ipso facto* increases the costs of restricting noncoital or collaborative reproduction by an unspecified but significant factor. Rights are therefore different from interests only in degree, not in kind.

This observation points to a second way in which Robertson's analysis is illuminating. His work allows us to see clearly the dangers of conflating a discussion of the legal status of assisted reproduction with that of its moral nature. That Robertson fails to distinguish legal issues from moral ones is clear throughout his writings, I believe, but it is most evident when he transposes the framework of balancing interests and costs from a legal context to a moral one. Robertson's discussion of the legal and ethical issues in human egg donation is a nice case in point. He begins his analysis of egg donation by invoking the familiar framework of compelling state interest vs. reproductive rights. He argues here, as elsewhere, that the right to procreate includes the right to procreate noncoitally and col-laboratively and that this right places the burden of proof on the state if it seeks to restrict access to assisted reproduction, in this case access to collaborative reproduction through the use of donor eggs. If the state is to restrict egg donation, it must demonstrate that collaborative reproduction through egg donation causes substantial harm. This, says Robertson, is something the state will not be able to do. If anything, egg donation "creates a more stable rearing and family situation" than other forms of collaborative reproduction because the rearing mother is also the gestation-al mother. Thus, there is a biological as well as social connection between mother and child, although there is no genetic connection.[26] So the state should not prohibit egg donation. Indeed, according to Robertson, states should facilitate egg donation by reducing uncertainties about rearing rights and duties in these cases and by allowing the providers of eggs to be paid for their services.

At this point, Robertson begins to blur the line between the moral assessment of egg donation and its legal status. Even if it is true that a right to procreate collaboratively is constitutionally protected and that states may not prohibit paying egg providers, it does not follow that allowing the sale of human ova is morally acceptable. Unfortunately, Robertson treats these issues as comparable. In keeping with his legal framework, Robert-son points out that there may be moral objections to paying women for ova, but opposition of this sort, he says, does not rise to the level of a compelling interest that would justify state intervention. Yet, again, it does not follow that since there is no compelling legal justification for prevent-ing the sale of ova, there is no compelling moral justification for so doing. Still, Robertson appears to think that determining the moral status of commercial egg transfer programs is essentially comparable to the process of weighing competing interests by undertaking a cost-benefit analysis. "The ethical objections to payment," he writes, "must be balanced against the need to pay women to assure an egg supply for needy recipients and to treat donors fairly."[27]

Despite the introduction of the language of fairness here, the moral calculus appears to follow the legal one. If the needs of the recipients are strong enough, the benefits they will receive from commercial egg transfer programs will simply outweigh the costs to the opponents who worry about the threat to human dignity created by such practices. Unfortunately, to say that the moral objections to the sale of human ova must be balanced against the need to maintain a steady supply for eager recipients is a bit like saying that the moral objections to slavery must be balanced against the need to bring in the cotton. In saying this I do not mean to suggest that the sale of human ova is morally comparable to the sale of human beings. Rather, the point is that moral deliberation is not always reducible to the sort of simple calculus Robertson utilizes in his analysis of the legal status of assisted reproduction.

Regrettably, this is not the only place in his writings that Robertson makes this mistake. In discussing the morality of aborting fetuses to acquire fetal tissue for transplants, Robertson is even more explicit in framing the moral question in essentially legal terms. Once again he moves from discussion of individual rights versus state interests to a moral conclusion based on balancing competing interests. Although aborting the fetus to obtain tissue does not harm the fetus, he says:

> it may impose symbolic costs measurable in terms of the reduced respect for human life generally that a willingness to abort early fetuses connotes. Still, the abortion may be ethically acceptable if the good sought sufficiently outweighs the symbolic devaluation of life that occurs when fetuses that cannot be harmed in their own right are aborted.[28]

Although Robertson is not here talking about issues in assisted reproduction, he makes the same argument in relation to using preimplantation embryos as he does for aborting embryos for tissue transplants. "The benefits of symbolizing respect by restricting activities with preimplantation embryos need to be weighed against the costs of doing so, and a policy judgment thus made on that basis."[29] Indeed, Robertson's treatment of the preimplantation embryo helps us to see both how thoroughly the legal framework of balancing individual rights and state interests shapes his discussion of the morality of assisted reproduction and how narrowly (and thus misleadingly) this framework construes the moral issues at stake in assisted reproduction.

Consider once again Robertson's claims about the preimplantation embryo. I agree with him that the preembryo is not a bearer of rights. In my view, the organism is not sufficiently developed at this stage to speak meaningfully about a being with rights. To be sure, the cells that constitute the early zygote or blastocyst are human, they are alive, they have the potential to develop into an adult human being, a bearer of rights. Yet these cells are still only very loosely organized and they are largely un-differentiated. They may still split to form two individuals or fuse to form less than one. There are as yet no structures identifiable as precursors to what would later be neural pathways or the brain. The early zygote or blastocyst cannot feel pain. It cannot fear death. It cannot experience anything at all. Indeed, even its potential at this point is significantly less than that of an implanted embryo only slightly more mature, for we know that both in nature and in the lab the chances of implantation for the zygote are not great, by any means. So I agree with Robertson here. The pre-implantation embryo is not the sort of organism to which we can meaning-fully attribute a right to life.

I know that many will not agree with this conclusion. Yet, even if we do agree with Robertson about the status of the preembryo, we may question the conclusions he draws about appropriate treatment of this organism. Why should we conclude from the fact that the preimplantation embryo is not a rights-bearing entity, that we can do with the preembryo more or less as we please? The reason Robertson draws this conclusion, I believe, is that he focuses his discussion almost exclusively in terms of the legal rights at stake in cases of fetal tissue transplants and assisted reproduction. Moreover, although Robertson warns against thinking about preimplanta-tion embryos and assisted reproduction as one would about fetuses and abortion, he does precisely that himself. That is why he applies the same framework of analogies when discussing fetal tissue transplants as when discussing the cryopreservation of embryos, for example. The reasoning in both instances is essentially the same. The right to privacy is a con-stitutionally protected right that safeguards, among other things, the free-dom to make important life decisions about reproduction, unconstrained by governmental interference. Because the fetus is not a person under the law, and therefore not a bearer of rights, reproductive privacy includes the freedom to choose to have an abortion, to use fetal tissue for transplants, or to freeze or discard embryos as one sees fit.

In reasoning in this way, Robertson fails to distinguish between a right to privacy and a right to bodily autonomy. Of course, in passing over this distinction Robertson is simply following the Supreme Court's lead in *Roe v. Wade*, where Justice Blackmun secured the freedom to choose abortion on the right to privacy, as critics on both the left and the right have frequently complained. Nevertheless, there are good reasons for drawing a distinction between privacy and bodily autonomy, not the least of which is that, although Justice Blackmun located the right to abortion in an interest in privacy rather than autonomy, the real concern of the Court seems to have been to relieve women of gestational burdens and thus protect their bodily autonomy.[30] In fact, Robertson himself has noted that to anchor the right to abortion on interests other than safeguarding bodily integrity is "more expansive justification than is necessary" and that "a woman's strongest moral claim" for abortion "is to bodily freedom and evidence of gestational burdens."[31]

If the right to abortion is meant to protect bodily autonomy, it does not follow that women therefore have a right to create a fetus in order to abort it to obtain fetal tissue or that they have a right to control the disposition of embryos created or stored *in vitro*, for in neither case is bodily integrity threatened. The right to bodily autonomy is not equivalent to the right to unrestricted use of embryos or fetuses for one's reproductive (or other) purposes, although Robertson often talks as if these two were the same. For example, in an essay on fetal tissue transplants from which I have already quoted, Robertson compares an abortion to end an unwanted pregnancy to an abortion to obtain tissue to save another person's life. "There is no sound ethical basis for prohibiting *this* [latter] sacrifice of the fetus when its sacrifice to end an unwanted pregnancy or pursue other goals is permitted."[32]

Notice, however, that this conclusion follows only if one assumes that the right to bodily autonomy is the same as the right to treat the fetus as an object at one's disposal. That Robertson makes this assumption is even clearer when he moves from considering aborting an already conceived fetus to obtain tissue to a discussion of conceiving a fetus with the sole purpose of aborting it to obtain tissue. He acknowledges that there may be more resistance to the latter case than to the former, because conceiving in order to abort denotes a willingness to use the fetus as a mere means in the service of one's ends, but he dismisses this concern as inconsistent. "Aborting when already pregnant to procure tissue for transplant *(or aborting for the more customary reasons)* also denotes a willingness to use the fetus as a means to other ends."[33] Thus Robertson equates aborting to protect bodily integrity (i.e., the customary reason) with aborting to obtain fetal tissue for transplant and with conceiving with the intention of aborting to obtain fetal tissue for transplant. He does so because he equates the right to bodily autonomy with the right to use the fetus as an object.

But why suppose that these two things are equivalent? Why suppose that aborting to avoid the physical burdens of gestation is to use the fetus as a means to one's ends? Narrowly construed, the right to bodily autonomy would only justify removing the fetus from one's body, not killing the fetus. Admittedly, in the early stages of pregnancy, as technology now stands, to remove a fetus from a woman's body is to kill the fetus and thus arguably to use the fetus to serve one's ends.[34] But terminating a pregnancy and terminating the life of the fetus are theoretically distinct and may become ever more practically so as technology develops. If we distinguish a right to bodily autonomy, understood as a right to avoid unwanted violations of bodily integrity, from some expansive right to use or to kill the fetus, there is a significant difference between aborting to end an unwanted pregnancy and aborting to obtain tissue for transplant, and there may well be a sound ethical basis for allowing the one and not the other.

Unfortunately, this failure to distinguish aborting to end an unwanted pregnancy and aborting to obtain tissue for transplants has implications for Robertson's discussion of assisted reproduction, for, as I noted above, he employs the same framework of analysis in discussing the use of embryos in assisted reproduction as he does their use in tissue transplants. In both cases, he assumes that the right to procreative autonomy protects the freedom to use the fetus as one sees fit. We have just seen, however, that a right to bodily autonomy does not entail such a guarantee. Why, then, does Robertson make this assumption?

The answer to this question, I believe, is that Robertson combines a commitment to bodily autonomy with a (largely undefended) view of the embryo and early fetus as mere tissue. That this is in fact Robertson's view of the embryo may not be clear at first because he frequently distinguishes various views of the status of the embryo and appears to reject the view that identifies the fetus as nothing more than ordinary human tissue. Yet, if we consider the alternatives here, we discover that this is, in effect, his view. According to Robertson, the three significant positions on the status of the embryo are these: (1) The embryo is a person with rights from conception (the embryo-as-person view); (2) The embryo is not a person and, indeed, is no different from any other human tissue (the embryo-as-tissue view); and (3) The embryo is not a person but deserves more respect than mere human tissue (the embryo-as-symbol view). Robertson explicitly rejects (1), implicitly denies (2), and appears to accept (3).[35]

At first blush, the dissimilarity between (2) and (3) would appear to underwrite significant differences in the treatment of human embryos. In the embryo-as-tissue view, the embryo is really no different from any other human tissue and thus deserves no special treatment. Consequently, in this view, treatment of the embryo should be left to the discretion of those whose tissue it is, i.e., the gamete providers, and there should be few, if any, restrictions on the use or disposal of embryos. By contrast, the embryo-as-symbol view appears to support very different conclusions. According to this view, although the embryo is not yet a person, it is nevertheless a potential person and therefore a potent symbol of human life. As a symbol of the human being the embryo deserves respect. While it may not be accorded the same status as a being with rights, it deserves to be treated differently from mere tissue. We are thus, within limits, fully justified in restricting what can and cannot be done to the embryo. So the embryo-as-tissue view appears to support nonintervention, whereas the embryo-as-symbol perspective appears to justify intervention.

This is not, however, the conclusion Robertson reaches. Although he apparently accepts the view of the fetus as a potential person symbolic of human life generally, he does not accept the corresponding restrictions on the use and disposal of embryos that such a perspective grounds. Indeed, as we have seen, while Robertson is typically suspicious of interventions to regulate assisted reproduction, he is especially insistent on rejecting those proposed for controlling the disposition of preimplantation embryos on symbolic grounds. Here we see how completely the narrow legal framework of individual rights versus state interests dominates his thinking. Although Robertson acknowledges the importance of a symbolic commitment to human life, this commitment is so thoroughly trumped by the procreative rights with which it may conflict that the harm of abandoning this commitment will not, in his view, justify opposition to assisted reproduction. Thus, for all practical purposes, the embryo-as-symbol view collapses into the embryo-as-tissue view, for in both cases, whatever is said about it, the embryo is *treated* as little more than simple tissue.

I believe it is a mistake to collapse these two perspectives on the embryo in this way, and one of the reasons I believe that Robertson makes this mistake is precisely that he is so preoccupied with the framework of individual (legal) rights. It is as if Robertson believes that because the embryo is not a rights-bearing entity, there is nothing left for it to be other than property. And if the embryo is property, it has no legal (or moral?) claim on us and deserves our attention only to the extent that its use or disposal conflicts with the rights of those who are fully persons.[36] This single-minded attention to legal rights is even evident in the cost-benefit analysis that Robertson argues justifies most reproductive interventions. We have seen that in weighing benefits and burdens the protection of rights counts as substantial benefit; it is also the case that both costs and benefits are defined almost exclusively in terms of rights. The benefits that flow from assisted reproduction are thus seen in terms of the satisfaction of those interests protected by the right to procreative autonomy, and the costs are measured in terms of the harm caused by interventions in the reproductive process. But, as we have seen, Robertson calculates harm in relation to rights, which is one reason he does not treat the possibility of serious harm to offspring as a significant cost of reproductive technology.

This preoccupation with rights perhaps makes sense if one is engaged in a strictly legal analysis of the status of assisted reproduction, but it is hard to defend as the sole basis of a moral analysis of reproductive technology, something Robertson also purports to offer. Consider, for example, the case just mentioned: Robertson's discussion of the possibility of harming off-spring through the use of novel reproductive techniques. It may well be the case that an analysis of the legal status of assisted reproduction requires us to draw a distinction between avoidable and unavoidable harm and to conclude, with Robertson, that because cases of unavoidable harm would not meet the traditional standards of tort liability—since no counterfactual comparison of the plaintiff's condition is possible—states are not justified in restricting reproductive technology to protect offspring from harm. Yet the fact that reproductive interventions may cause damage that does not meet the legal definition of harm, or that parents cannot be said to have a legal obligation to refrain from conceiving in certain ways or under certain circumstances, does not mean that we are morally free to do as we like here. Parents bear a responsibility for their children that supervenes any legal obligation to avoid harm. Indeed, as I suggested in chapter 2, we must reject Derek Parfit's account of harm. It just does not matter morally that a woman who knowingly conceives a defective child would not have conceived the same child had she waited several months to avoid foreseeable harm. To rely on this reasoning to say that she has not harmed the child she conceives is sophistry. So, too, should we reject the equally anemic view of harm that allows Robertson to say that the greatest harm of transferring embryos possibly damaged by research manipulations is to those who "end up bearing the costs of caring for handicapped off-spring."

Toward a More Expansive View of Responsible Reproduction

In short, we need a much more expansive vision of the commitments and obligations that constrain morally responsible interventions in the reproductive process. There are more ways to act badly in pursuing parenthood than are dreamed of in Robertson's narrowly legalistic treatment of assisted reproduction. In part, the problem facing Robertson's analysis is the same one we noted in chapter 2 when we discussed the analogy between sexual prostitution and reproductive prostitution. In a political milieu that stresses individual fulfillment and that defines liberty as freedom from interference by others, it is difficult to frame a public policy that takes account of the common good and is prepared to accept some tradeoff between individual liberty and social responsibility.

Moreover, even if we accept Robertson's concentration on an analysis of the legal rights at stake in assisted reproduction, we may question his particular interpretation of these rights. Recall that for Robertson rights are correlated with interests and that he identifies at least three distinct interests in procreation. Individuals have an interest in genetic parenthood, gestational parenthood, and social parenthood. This is why he says that full procreative freedom would include the right to separate the genetic, gestational, and rearing aspects of procreation and to recombine them in collaboration with others.[37] Yet we may acknowledge that individuals typically do have an interest in all three components of procreation when they reproduce and still question whether the interest in any one component isolated from the others is protected by a right to procreative autonomy. Robertson himself acknowledges that there may well be limits to constitutionally protected liberties when the components of reproduction are disaggregated, but he never conducts the sort of analysis of the individual and social goods at stake in procreation that would allow us to establish the moral or legal boundaries of these liberties.[38]

However, because Robertson does not undertake this sort of analysis and because his discussion of the right to procreate follows very closely his reading of the Court cases establishing a right not to procreate, Robertson understands the right to procreative autonomy largely as a right to use one's body—or another's with consent—in whatever way one chooses to produce genetic offspring, at least if one plans to rear the resulting off-spring. Just as the right not to procreate leaves one free to separate sex from procreation, so does the right to procreate leave one free to procreate without sex, or in collaboration with others, or by design through genetic screening, etc., so long as one produces genetic offspring that one will rear. Yet Robertson never really asks whether the interest in having and rearing genetic descendants is an interest of such central social value that it ought to be protected at almost any cost. We must ask the question Robertson fails to ask: Do we really want to endorse, either morally or legally, the overriding value of genetic connection?

Certainly, we can acknowledge the value of having and rearing biological descendants, both to individuals and to society. Certainly, too, for the typical infertile couple the desire for children will be a desire for off-spring genetically related to both partners. As Leon Kass has pointed out, a couple's desire for a family is probably best captured in a rather archaic idiom that nevertheless expresses the force of biological connection. "The desire to have a child of one's own," he writes, "is a *couple's* desire to embody, out of the conjugal union of their separate bodies, a child who is flesh of their separate flesh made one."[39] I would be the last person to deny the importance and power of this desire. As my wife and I confronted our continuing infertility, the emotion we felt most acutely was that of loss over the child we had believed we would have together. It was the desire literally to embody our love, more than any other desire, that led us to endure the painful tests, the surgery, the loss of control, and the cycle of hope and despair that is part of infertility treatment. Those who have been helped by reproductive technology to embody their love know the fulfill-ment that comes from the satisfaction of this desire, even when the cost is high. So I will not discount the importance of this desire.

At the same time, however, we must ask about the price that is paid if we elevate the desire for genetic offspring to the status of a legally or morally privileged interest. Barbara Katz Rothman, for example, has pointed out that while the desire for genetic connection is important, in our culture it often reflects and reinforces a patriarchal view of the family.[40] It reflects a patriarchal system because, under patriarchy, paternity is the central social relationship and genetic ties are the fundamental basis of reckoning kinship. A preoccupation with paternity may thus underlie a desire for genetic connection because, in the absence of this connection, members of a household may not be considered really related. In the absence of genetic ties, questions may persist about who the "real" father and the "real" mother are.[41] Under these circumstances, it should not be surprising to discover that couples are willing to undergo a great deal to conceive genetically related offspring, and this, in turn, works to reinforce a commitment to the centrality of genetic connection, for the message is quite clear: genetic connection must be important, otherwise no one would be willing to endure such significant sacrifices in its pursuit.

Rothman nicely captures this dialectic in a passage worth quoting at some length:

> Out of our beliefs, values, and ideas we create social structure and social institutions. And then those institutions reify our ideology. We believe, for example, that genetic ties are the real ties, the only permanent, irreducible connections. And then we create a world in which those ties are indeed valued, recognized, and attended to—made real socially. Paternity based on a single sexual encounter stands on the same legal ground as the paternity of a loving husband and father, a man committed for the long haul. And that recognition of a man's genetic tie at the same time undercuts the recognition and support of his social, emotional, and nurturing ties. *Paternity* has more social support than has *fathering*. Our beliefs about genetics similarly limit the ways we can think about infertility, with some solutions seen as real, and some as alternatives, second best, making do. And so we create social structures that reinforce those beliefs: the modern creation of the anonymous adoption, the "matched" child substituting for the "real" child.[42]

Rothman's observation here about how a belief in the superiority of genetic connection, reinforced by social institutions, structures the choices in infertility treatment dovetails with our discussion in chapter 2 about the way in which the very existence of reproductive technology generates inescapable but unwanted choices. More important, Rothman draws our attention to the way in which concern about genetic connection may lead us to neglect the importance of loving, nurturing relationships in the constitution of a family. In Rothman's words, nurturance matters "more than genetics, loving more than lineage, and care more than kinship."[43] Unfortunately, the presuppositions of modern reproductive technology are frequently the reverse.

We can see the price paid for this reversal by attending to how differently an approach that emphasizes individual rights and that treats the embryo as quasi-property owned by its genetic parents is from one that assigns a more central place to relationships than to rights and that treats the embryo as more than mere tissue. Both will readily approve of the sort of reproductive interventions that we considered in the first two chapters. Both AIH and the simplest applications of IVF will, in general, promote reproductive autonomy without sacrificing social, emotional, or nurturing ties. But now consider the extensions of assisted reproduction discussed in this chapter. Focusing primarily on individual rights and the pursuit of private procreative interests, Robertson finds little difficulty extending the logic that justifies AIH and IVF to the justification of cryopreservation of human embryos, manipulations of embryos and gametes for eugenic purposes, collaborative reproduction in a variety of forms, and even the commercialization of reproduction. Given the focus on individual rights, so long as the participants in assisted reproduction consent to the activities in which they are engaged, and so long as no one is substantially harmed who has not consented to these activities, there is scarcely a reason not to accept every extension of reproductive technology.

By contrast, if one does not focus exclusively on individual rights or measure success solely in terms of reproducing one's genes, things look quite different. One is freed, for example, to ask questions that do not readily occur when attention is focused on individual rights. Instead of asking: will someone's rights be violated by thus and so an intervention? we may ask: will this reproductive intervention affect the establishment of a deep and lasting emotional bond between parent and child? Instead of: are there compelling state interests to justify restricting individual freedom? we ask: how may the state facilitate the nurturing relationships between adults and children that are so crucial to both individual and social well-being?

It was a question of this latter sort that I attempted to press in chapter 1 when I asked how the high costs of assisted reproduction might shape our attitudes toward the children produced in this manner. Indeed, in my view only an impoverished account of moral responsibility would preclude us from asking these sorts of questions. Yet when we ask, for example, about the impact of assisted reproduction, and especially about the impact of those forms engendered by cryopreservation of embryos and collaborative reproduction, on our attitudes toward children or toward women—when we ask whether assisted reproduction helps promote or perhaps frustrates the nurturance necessary to children's well-being—it becomes difficult to give the sort of wholesale endorsement of assisted reproduction that Robertson offers. His affirmation of the right to control the characteristics of offspring through the genetic alteration of embryos, his defense of the right of parents to control the disposition of frozen embryos, including the right to use them for tissue transplants or for research purposes, his acceptance of the right to sell embryos and gametes to facilitate full procreative autonomy—all seem strangely unreflective of the possibility that to exercise these rights may not be good for parents or for children or for the relationship between parents and children.

In short, if we do not restrict our discussion of the morality of assisted reproduction to an analysis of the rights of the various participants in the process, we are much less likely to give unqualified approval to reproductive interventions. This is not to say that to ask questions about relationships as well as about rights is to oppose assisted reproduction altogether. We saw in the first chapter, for example, that to be concerned that the expense of assisted reproduction may lead us to treat our children as costly investments rather than priceless gifts does not necessarily lead to the conclusion that assisted reproduction ought to be morally resisted. On the contrary, I argued that, despite the cost, AIH and the simplest cases of IVF are morally acceptable. Still, to raise concerns about how interventions in the reproductive process may affect the way parents relate to children or children to parents or about how assisted reproduction may lead us to think about women's role in reproduction, and to be prepared to reject reproductive interventions that adversely affect women or children, is to proceed much more cautiously in respect of extensions of basic reproductive technology than Robertson does.

Our discussion of the limitations of Robertson's approach, then, leads us to see the need for finding a middle way between the unqualified rejection of reproductive technology described in chapter 1 and the almost unqualified acceptance described in this chapter. I hope it is also now clear that the fact that I argued against the one (unqualified rejection) is not evidence that I accept the other (unqualified acceptance). To disagree with the Vatican that all forms of assisted reproduction are morally repugnant is not to agree with Robertson that all forms are morally salutary. This is particularly evident when attention is focused on collaborative reproduction, for although many are prepared, against the teaching of the Vatican, to accept noncollaborative interventions, far fewer are willing, with Robertson, to embrace collaborative reproduction wholeheartedly.

The topic of collaborative reproduction thus provides fertile ground, so to speak, for an investigation of the proper boundaries of morally acceptable interventions in the reproductive process. If we are to find a middle road between unqualified acceptance and unqualified rejection, it is likely to cut a path through the various forms of collaborative reproduction. Artificial insemination with donor sperm, *in vitro* fertilization with donor eggs, surrogate motherhood, gestational surrogacy, and embryo adoption all involve intimate third party collaboration in the reproductive process, and each forces us to address the question of whether, and under what circumstances, it is morally acceptable to divide up genetic, gestational, and social parenthood. It is to this question, then, that I turn in the next two chapters, as I seek to mark the way between the extreme positions on assisted reproduction.

Part II

Defining Parenthood

THE CHALLENGE OF REPRODUCTIVE
TECHNOLOGY

4

Donor Insemination and Responsible Parenting

> Gentlemen of the jury, what is a father—a
> real father . . .?
>   How shall it be decided? Why, like this.
> Let the son stand before the father and
> ask him, "Father, tell me why I must love
> you? Father, show that I must love you,"
> and if that father is able to answer him
> and show him good reason, we have a
> real, normal, parental relation, not resting
> on mystical prejudice [for genetic connec-
> tion], but on a rational, responsible and
> strictly humanitarian basis. But if he does
> not, there's an end to the family tie.
> —*The Brothers Karamazov.*[1]

To this point, my position on assisted reproduction has been defined largely in relation to the extremes. On the one hand, I have rejected the view that virtually every intervention in the reproductive process is harmful and ought to be avoided. On the other hand, I have dismissed claims to the effect that individuals have an overriding right to procreate with whomever and by whatever means they choose, even where the consequences to the children so produced are unknown or unfortunate. To survey the boundaries of a defensible position on assisted reproduction, however, is not to have a complete lay of the land. To know what you reject is not necessarily to know what you accept, and it is always easier to criticize than to offer a constructive alternative.

This chapter and the next, then, take up the task of developing a more constructive position on assisted reproduction than I have hitherto presented. Our discussions of AIH and IVF have provided a useful introduction to many of the moral issues raised by reproductive technology, but because neither AIH nor the cases of IVF on which I have focused have involved third-party collaborators, we have not had to confront several questions central to the project of articulating a coherent and nuanced position on assisted reproduction. For example, we have not addressed the

71

question of what it means to be a parent. Should parenthood be defined primarily in terms of genetic connections, or should it be defined socially? What goods or values do individuals seek to realize when they decide to become parents? What responsibilities flow from that decision? These questions arise almost immediately when we consider forms of collaborative reproduction that involve the contribution of third-party gametes, and, as we shall see, answering these sorts of questions takes us a good distance toward the completion of our project.

Donor Gametes and the Meaning of Parenthood

I turn first to discuss artificial insemination with donor sperm, for it was the availability of DI that forced my wife and me to confront the meaning of parenthood. As I indicated in the Introduction, we ultimately decided to try donor insemination, but this decision was not made quickly or easily. We talked about donor insemination for hours over many months. We decided almost immediately that if we did pursue DI we would do so openly, telling our family and close friends and, ultimately, our child. We met with psychologists to discuss the impact of such information on the development of a child's sense of identity. We worried about the asymmetry that donor insemination would pose in our relation to our child. Lisa would be both the genetic and social mother; I would be the social father but not the genetic father. How would this feel? How would it feel to watch Lisa grow with the child produced by another's sperm? How would it feel to hear others say that our child did not look like me or, indeed, that he did look like me? How would it feel to hear our child say—perhaps in rebellion during adolescence, but surely some time—that I was not his or her real father? Would I love such a child differently or less? I could go on.

We ultimately decided upon donor insemination because we believed that rearing a child most essentially defined the meaning of parenthood and that doing so together was, in the final analysis, what we sought in trying to become parents. To be sure, we had wanted literally to embody our love, to produce a child who might have Lisa's smile, say, and my eyes. But this desire to have a child of our "own" was not a desire for genetic offspring; it was a desire for our union in a child. And if we could not have a child that was the result of our physical union, we could have a child that was the product of our spiritual union, who might also happen to have Lisa's smile. More important, we believed we could love this child unconditionally. Such a child would place special demands on its parents—and we tried hard not to deceive ourselves about these—but every child places special demands on its parents. Certainly this is true of an adopted child, and at the time we were deciding about DI, that was our other choice.

This chapter, then, is in part a defense of our decision. I ask, in a different context and in a different voice, whether we were right to define parenthood primarily in social terms. Obviously, I believe that we were right and that there are very good reasons for defining parenthood socially. Nevertheless, this remains a controversial claim, and the practice of DI remains a controversial practice.[2]

It may thus be useful to begin by asking why donor insemination is so controversial. This fact may at first be surprising, for DI is typically used in cases like mine, as an alternative treatment of male infertility, when AIH has failed. Yet AIH is not controversial. As we have seen, almost no one questions the morality of AIH, and although the Catholic church has raised concerns about it, even the Vatican is prepared to accept AIH when it is not a substitute for sexual intercourse. Both procedures are simple, both involve laboratory preparation of semen, both involve the implantation of semen into the vagina or uterus. So why is there a different moral response to DI?

The answer, of course, is related to the central difference between DI and AIH. With donor insemination, semen is typically provided anonymously by a third party, whereas with AIH semen comes from the spouse of the woman inseminated. Should this difference underwrite a corresponding difference in our moral judgments about AIH and DI? A substantial number of thoughtful commentators have argued that it should. When we examine why, we are led back to concerns about the meaning of marriage and parenthood. Leon Kass is fairly typical in this regard. We saw in chapter 3 that Kass is prepared to accept some forms of assisted reproduction, but not interventions that involve third parties. In Kass's view, the problem with DI, and other forms of collaborative reproduction involving third parties, is that they separate genetic, gestational, and social parenthood and thus weaken as well as obscure the bonds of lineage, kinship, and descent. The problem with weakening those bonds is that they are central to individual and social stability. Kass's vision of the consequences of weakening these bonds is apocalyptic indeed. In language that could not but conjure images of a holocaust, Kass asks, "Are we to accept as desirable the *final solution* that eliminates biological kinship from the foundation of social organization?"[3]

Although I do not agree with the importance Kass places on genetic kinship and lineage, nor with the conclusion he draws that civilized society would be threatened by widespread use of collaborative reproduction, I believe that Kass is at least asking the right questions. His claims about the importance of genetic connection emerge in the context of a discussion about what it means "to have a child of one's own." That is, Kass asks precisely those questions that need to be asked: What does it mean to decide to become a parent? Is genetic or social parenthood more important? What benefits do we seek in pursuing parenthood?

Unfortunately, in answering these questions Kass draws a sharp distinction between those aspects or dimensions of parenthood that involve physically and emotionally nurturing a child and those that involve the physical generation of children. He poses a stark either/or. Is the crucial meaning of having a child of one's own "to nourish and to rear, the child being the embodiment of one's activity as teacher and guide"? "Or is it rather," he writes, "to provide someone who descends and comes after, someone who will replace oneself in the family line or preserve the family tree by new sproutings and branchings, someone who will renew and perpetuate the vitality and aspiration of human life?"[4] Yet why suppose that our answer to the question of what it means to be a parent involves an exclusive choice? Why suppose that in affirming the importance of rearing a child, we must deny the importance of genetic connection? To be sure, when a couple confronts the decision whether to pursue DI, they must decide whether physically and emotionally nurturing a child who is genetically related to only one of them will accomplish what they seek to accomplish in having children.[5] But the fact that a couple may answer yes here does not mean that they dismiss the *relative* significance of genetic connection. Indeed, I fail to see why someone who was willing to accept DI to overcome infertility could not say with Kass that he sought precisely "to renew and perpetuate the vitality and aspiration of human life."

In fairness to Kass, he does not say that in trying to have a child of their own a couple seeks simply to pass on their genes. If that were the case, you would not expect to find any sense of loss, for example, in a case of DI where the husband's identical twin is the donor. Yet, as Kass correctly points out, this would not be a matter of indifference to the couple.[6] Surely Kass is right about this, and he may well be right that the language that best captures the desire of the couple is traditional and somewhat archaic, that the desire is "to embody, out of the conjugal union of their separate bodies, a child who is flesh of their separate flesh made one."[7] As I mentioned, this language certainly captures something of my experience. So I would not deny the importance of the experience to which Kass draws our attention here.

Yet we should not just assume, as Kass does, that genetic connection is constitutive of parenthood. Because Kass assumes that parenthood is defined by genetic connection, he sees parenthood without genetic connection as potentially disastrous. But if genetic connection is of overriding significance, this should be the conclusion, not the starting point, of Kass's discussion of what it means to have a child of one's own. Even if we grant that would-be parents ideally desire to create a child who is flesh of their flesh, this is not all they desire in pursuing parenthood. They seek as well to establish a relationship with a child whom they will nourish and nurture, teach and train. Indeed, Kass himself admits that one might desire a child who is the embodiment "of one's own activity as teacher and guide." Yet he fails to realize that a child may be the embodiment of a couple's love and care in a sense that is every bit as real as the embodiment of their love in the physical sense that he is flesh of their flesh.

That Kass sees only one of these loves as truly embodied is revealed in his remark that assisted reproduction involving third parties is degrading and dehumanizing because it is a "blind assertion of will against our bodily nature," a comment that reveals a blindness to the fact that caring for children—however they are conceived—is no mere assertion of the will, but is a bodily affair from start to finish. Indeed, when Kass talks here about individuals using their bodies as mere tools in undertaking third-party–assisted reproduction, he ignores the fact that DI is typically undertaken in a context in which what is sought is precisely the physical embodiment of love in a child. (And as we have seen there is more than one way to embody love in a child.) DI no more challenges the meaning of embodiment, is no more a blind assertion of will, than is any other effort to overcome physical (embodied) obstacles to the realization of our willful projects. Walking with a prosthetic leg does not challenge the meaning of embodiment, nor does taking platelets to control coagulation, nor does undergoing reconstructive tubal surgery. I am not saying that undergoing DI is the same as any of these, morally speaking. Rather, my point is that, *in terms of what each implies about embodiment,* they are the same. On the contrary, the need in each case to correct physical imperfections is a potent reminder of the meaning of embodiment. Is DI really so different from these?

The answer to this question depends on how one views the relationship between the values sought in overcoming the bodily obstacles to having children and the means of overcoming these obstacles. In the case of prosthetic devices, supplemental clotting factor, or tuboplasty, the means of correcting physical impairment does not fundamentally alter the nature of the good or value desired. Can we say the same of DI? Presumably, Kass's discussion of what it means to have a child of one's own was an attempt to answer this question. Yet, as we have seen, because Kass assumes that genetic connection is of primary importance, the question is obscured rather than answered. We therefore need to ask the question again: What does it mean to have a child of one's own? What precisely do individuals/couples seek when they decide to become parents? And more to the point: If individuals or couples seek more than one goal in pursuing parenthood, how should we approach the case where these goals or values are separated, either accidentally or intentionally? Is the meaning of parenthood so transformed in such a case that we no longer acknowledge the goal pursued here as a worthy one?

We can begin by noting that the desire to become a parent, the desire to have a child of one's own, is extremely complex and is rarely just one desire. Nevertheless, the various desires involved in pursuing parenthood can be sorted according to the goals toward which they move. For example, in *Reproductive Ethics,* Michael Bayles proposes that the desire to have children will take one of three forms: the desire to beget, to bear, or to rear a child. To his three types I would add a fourth, namely, the desire to beget a child with another. Pursuing parenthood may thus involve the desire (a) to pass on one's genes, (b) to embody one's love for another in a child who is the result of the physical union with one's beloved, (c) to carry and to nurture a child in one's body, or (d) to lovingly bring up a child.[8] Of course, in most cases pursuing parenthood will involve a combination of these desires, for in seeking genetic, gestational, or social parenthood, individuals or couples generally try to realize or to give expression to a variety of aspirations. In pursuing parenthood we may seek a sort of immortality, affirm commitment to a spouse, express hope in the future, or ensure sexual identity or a sense of adulthood. And these aspirations may be realized in different ways in relation to the genetic, gestational, and rearing components of parenthood. Still, we face the question, How should we think about the case where the genetic, gestational, and social forms of parenthood are separated, either accidentally or intentionally?

The Accidental Separation of Genetic and Social Parenthood: The Case of Kimberly Mays

Let us take the case of inadvertent separation first. Admittedly, these cases will be uncommon, for they involve an unlikely scenario in which genetic parenthood is split from gestational or social parenthood without the knowledge or consent of the gestational or social parents.[9] Either a woman unknowingly carries and raises a child who is not genetically related to her, or she unknowingly raises a child different from the one she carried and to whom she gave birth. The first case might result from a mix-up of embryos during an IVF procedure, the second from an accidental misidentification of children in a hospital nursery. Neither is very likely, and so such cases will indeed be rare. Still, they happen and they can be instructive.

Consider, for example, a case that received national media attention in the fall of 1988. The case involved two couples, Ernest and Regina Twigg and Robert and Barbara Mays, whose biological children had apparently been switched at birth, nine years earlier. The mistake was discovered during the summer of 1988, shortly before the Twiggs' daughter, Arlena, died of complications from surgery she had undergone to repair a congenital heart defect. In the course of medical treatment leading up to surgery, the Twiggs learned that Arlena was blood type B, although they were both blood type O. Concerned by this inconsistency, the Twiggs had tests run at the immunogenetics lab at Johns Hopkins University. These tests revealed that Arlena was not their biological daughter.

The Twiggs then hired a private investigator and a lawyer and discovered that another girl had been born in the same hospital at approximately the same time as Arlena to Barbara and Robert Mays. The Twiggs concluded that the girls had been switched in the hospital, and they filed a $100 million lawsuit against the hospital and sought a court order to have Robert Mays's nine-year-old daughter, Kimberly, undergo genetic testing to determine if she was their biological child.[10] Subsequently, the FBI investigated the case and found no evidence of criminal misconduct, and the Twiggs agreed not to seek custody if Robert Mays would allow Kimberly to undergo genetic testing. Mays agreed, and the tests showed that Kimberly was in fact the Twiggs' biological offspring.

What lessons may we draw about the meaning of parenthood from this case? The case appears to pose precisely the sort of either/or choice that I suggested frames Kass's discussion of the possibility of dividing parenthood. That is, we are initially inclined to ask: Who are Kimberly's parents, the Twiggs or the Mayses? Is Kimberly's father Ernest Twigg or Robert Mays? Such questions are understandable because genetic and social parenthood ordinarily go together. Moreover, when they are accidentally separated, as in this case, we are likely to think that the genetic parents have been regrettably deprived of something to which they have a claim, and so when the Twiggs seek to have Kimberly tested genetically or when they seek custody or visitation rights, we may be initially sympathetic. Yet we can (and should) acknowledge the sense of shock the Twiggs must have felt to discover that Arlena was not their biological child, and we can (and should) understand their curiosity to know whether Kimberly is their biological child, without assuming with Kass that genetic connection provides the Twiggs with a privileged parental claim. I believe this case helps us to see precisely why Kass is mistaken in his approach to the meaning of parenthood. Consider what Kass's view would lead us to conclude about this case. If parenthood should be defined primarily in terms of genetic connection, if social stability requires us to privilege genetic kinship, then the Twiggs really do have a parental claim that trumps any other. The Twiggs should be declared Kimberly's legal parents, and they should be awarded custody, with visitation rights for Robert Mays to be left to their discretion. In other words, Kass's approach forces us to ask who the "real" parents are here, and given his emphasis on the importance of genetic kinship, he cannot but answer that Ernest and Regina Twigg are Kimberly's "real" parents.

Unfortunately, any talk about the "real" parents in such a case is likely to be profoundly misleading because it will incline us to deny some reality. To say that Ernest Twigg is Kimberly's "real" father is to deny the reality of ten years of genuine fatherly care and concern by Robert Mays. To say that Robert Mays is Kimberly's "real" father is to deny the reality that Kimberly is Ernest Twigg's biological offspring. There is, however, one sense in which asking who Kimberly's "real" father is may be enlightening rather than misleading. If we understand this question to embody a recognition that Kimberly has more than one father and to be a shorthand way of asking, of the various ways in which Kimberly has been fathered, which do we wish to assign the greatest importance, then this question may usefully focus our discussion. Notice that, understood in this way, the question does not presuppose an either/or answer. Rather, it is a question that asks us to weigh the respective parental activities undertaken by Ernest Twigg and Robert Mays and to assign them an importance relative to one another.

If this is what it means to ask who Kimberly's "real" parents are, then the answer that would follow from Kass's discussion is rather implausible. If we think of Ernest Twigg and Robert Mays as representing the distinct activities of begetting a child, on the one hand, and of raising a child, on the other, surely we will say that the latter is more important and that Robert Mays is Kimberly's father. And to say this is not to deny that Kimberly is Ernest Twigg's biological child. Rather, it is to say that responsible parenthood comprises a variety of activities and that, of those activities, nurturing and nourishing a child in the context of an ongoing social, emotional, and loving relationship is more important than physically begetting a child, however ineradicable and significant the physical/biological connection that is created thereby.

At the core of responsible parenthood is the commitment to, and the activities of, caring for a child in a way that promotes human flourishing.[11] Responsible parenthood thus involves nurturing, teaching, loving, and training a child in one's care. To be sure, responsible parenthood will often involve a decision to bring a child into existence, and the typical case will involve physically begetting a child as well. In my view, neither the intention nor the act of creating new life is essential.[12] Thus, there will be cases where responsible parenthood does not involve a decision to create a new life, but instead involves the decision to nurture a child who is not one's biological offspring. In short, it is the social relationship to a child that makes the parent, and while genetic connection may foster relational bonds, it is the bonds that are crucial, not the genetic ties.[13]

In arguing for the centrality of the relational bond between parent and child and in defending the primacy of Robert Mays's claim to parenthood, I am not suggesting that the Twiggs's relationship to Kimberly is trivial or insignificant. On the contrary, defining parenthood relationally rather than genetically allows us to be sympathetic and understanding both of the Twiggs' desire to know whether Kimberly is their biological daughter, and to know Kimberly, if she is, and of the possibility that Kimberly might desire to know the Twiggs. These desires are understandable because the Twiggs made a commitment to care for Kimberly, even if that commitment was unrealized, through no fault of their own. They have a link with Kimberly—and Kimberly with them—however tenuous that link may be. Kimberly is the person who embodies Ernest and Regina's love for one another, and the Twiggs had a direct, nurturing relationship with Kimberly, if only for the nine months of Regina's pregnancy. To be sure, the intensity and depth of that relationship does not compare to the intensity and depth of Robert Mays's relationship with Kimberly. Nevertheless, the Twiggs' connection to Kimberly is real and cannot be denied. So while I defend Robert Mays's rights and responsibilities as Kimberly's father, I also acknowledge the Twiggs' interest in Kimberly as understandable and legitimate.

We began our discussion of Kimberly's case with the hope that reflecting on a situation in which genetic and social parenthood had been inadvertently separated might help us to think more clearly about donor insemination, a case where genetic and social parenthood are not accidentally, but intentionally, separated. More specifically, we turned to this case with the question of whether the absence of a genetic connection between a "parent" and child so transforms the meaning of parenthood that we cannot value parenthood as fully in such a case as when a child is raised by his/her own genetic parent. I hope that our discussion has shown that as significant as genetic connection may be, it is the ongoing, caring relationship with a child that is the core of responsible parenthood. To repeat: parenthood is constituted primarily in relationship, not in genetic connection.[14] It follows that we can value an ongoing committed relationship to care as responsible parenthood, whether such a commitment is rooted in biological connection or not.

The Intentional Separation of Genetic and Social Parenthood

It is one thing to value the commitment of an adult to foster the growth and well-being of a child already in existence, irrespective of biological relation; it is quite another matter to affirm the creation of a child who will not be cared for by his or her biological parents. So even if we affirm the centrality of the caring relationship and thus the primacy of social parenthood in the case of adoption or accidental separation of genetic and social parenthood, we are left with a question: Is creating a child with the intention of separating moral and genetic parenthood morally acceptable? We must ask this question because it is possible to argue that while separating genetic and social parenthood may be commendable to ameliorate a situation in which a genetic parent cannot properly care for a child, it is never commendable to create the situation. The one case, it might be said, responds to an unfortunate set of circumstances; the other chooses these circumstances. This position has been vigorously defended by Lisa Sowle Cahill, and it is well worth reviewing her argument as we seek to answer the question posed above.

According to Cahill, there is a qualitative difference between forms of assisted reproduction that involve the use of third-party gametes—and thus separate genetic and social parenthood—and those that do not. The difference has to do with the moral significance of genetic connection. In Cahill's view, moral responsibilities are directly contingent upon the physical relation of genetic connection, and these responsibilities are essentially inalienable. So, for Cahill, the very existence of genetic connection is sufficient to ground moral obligations, and these obligations cannot be completely transferred to others. The upshot is that it could never be morally acceptable to create a child with the intention of separating genetic and social parenthood; to do so would require an individual to create a set of moral obligations he or she had no intention of discharging. Indeed, in this view, even adoption becomes somewhat morally uncertain. While it may be in the best interest of a child to set aside the obligations generated by genetic connection, in the final analysis, these obligations are ineradicable. Cahill writes:

> Even in the case of post-natal adoption, where birth parents are understood to have severed their ties to the child permanently, the statement of absolute relinquishment is in a sense a legal fiction put in place prudently to protect the "best interest" of the child and of the yielding parents as well. The immense interest of adopted children in discovering their biological "roots," and the frequent reciprocation by birth parents, however, testify to the fact that natural kinship bonds remain, whatever the intentions of individuals to step outside them. *Adoptive parents create real parental bonds, but these bonds may remain in an ambiguous moral (even if not legal) relationship to the natural bonds of the biological parents with the child.*[15]

In other words, parents who relinquish their biological children for adoption do not thereby eliminate their moral responsibilities to these children, nor presumably do they forfeit their rights. Whatever we may want to say about such cases legally, morally there are rights and responsibilities that cannot simply be willed out of existence.

This last point about intentionality is important because Cahill arrives at her position from a deep skepticism about a liberal commitment to autonomy and self-determination. In fact, Cahill develops her position in contradistinction to the work of Lori Andrews and Barbara Katz Rothman, both of whom emphasize the importance of individual choice in determining the responsibilities of parenthood. By contrast, for Cahill, "Parenthood is a relation whose existence cannot be made entirely contingent on choice."[16] She argues that "biological relationships can and should exercise some constraints upon freedom to choose (or not choose) the parental relation."[17] Among the freedoms that biological relation ought to constrain is the freedom to choose donor insemination and surrogate motherhood.

For Cahill there is a "natural" normative ideal of parenthood that ought to constrain the choices of infertile couples. In her view, sex, marriage, and parenthood have certain inner connections that should not be violated, except to avoid harm to a child. One of these connections is embodied in the parents' shared genetic relationship to the child. Consequently, to choose to procreate in a way that intentionally separates genetic and social parenthood is to violate the basic family structure by departing from the normative ideal. Since we should not intentionally violate this basic structure, the normative ideal serves to constrain individual choice.

Cahill appears to assume, however, that to allow individuals intentionally to separate social and genetic parenthood is to abandon all constraints on reproductive choice. Hence her comment that the relation of parenthood cannot be made entirely contingent on choice. It is as if Cahill sees the options as either accepting her normative ideal, thereby accepting restrictions on the means of reproducing, or else rejecting her ideal, thereby making parenthood entirely contingent on choice. These are not the only options here. The issue is not whether there is a normative ideal to which we must subject our will, but what form that ideal takes. For Cahill, having genetic and social parenthood together is at the core of her normative ideal; in my view, this is not part of the core. In disagreeing with Cahill about the normative ideal, I am not abandoning all restraints on reproductive choice. I am simply drawing the line of acceptable choice at a different place.

Nor is Cahill alone in suggesting that a view like mine makes the responsibilities of parenthood entirely contingent on choice. Responding to an earlier version of my argument, James Tunstead Burtchaell has suggested that I restrict, and thus reduce, the responsibilities of the parent-child relationship to ones that are freely chosen only. He thus attributes to me a conclusion, the patent absurdity of which he believes is enough to show the mistake of defining parenthood socially. According to Burtchaell, in arguing for the primacy of social relation as definitive of parenthood, I choose to privilege child-rearing rather than child-bearing, because the former "entails a social relation." "The clear implication," Burtchaell continues, "is that we are invested with no social relations except by acts of choice. This would imply that parents (purposeful parents) have a social relationship with their children but that children do not necessarily have a social relationship with their parents, because they never chose them."[18]

If this were the consequence of my view, I would indeed be worried. Fortunately, it is not. Contrary to Burtchaell's claim, I do not choose to emphasize child-rearing as opposed to child-bearing because child-rearing entails a social relation. The fact of social relation itself creates responsibilities, for the parent as well as for the child. Like Cahill, Burtchaell seeks to impose a false dichotomy. Either acknowledge the fact of genetic connection—and thus privilege a genetic definition of parenthood—or make parental responsibility entirely contingent on choice. Burtchaell describes his decision to report a suspected instance of foul play during a traffic accident. "My decision did not create my duty; it fulfilled it. I had either to embrace or to shirk an obligation whose existence and extent were created by facts, not choice."[19] Why does Burtchaell suppose that the same thing cannot be said of the responsibilities of a social father to his donor child? Jut as I would not say that children are freed of obligations to their parents because they did not freely choose the social relationship they have to their parents, so I would not say that parents are free of obligations to their children if they choose to ignore them.

Of course, parents can choose not to meet their responsibilities, and noting this fact may help us to appreciate one type of worry that could easily arise in relation to arguments like those of Burtchaell or Cahill. Let us return for a moment to Cahill's argument in order to identify this second sort of worry.

Although Cahill seeks nonconsequentialist grounds to oppose the use of third-party gametes, her argument is easily taken in a consequentialist direction. For example, one plausible interpretation of Cahill's basic concern here is that if we allow choice to determine where parental responsibilities begin, we will allow choice to determine where they end as well. Or to put the point more sharply: if we are free to create a parental relation with a child regardless of biological relation, we are free to sever that relation if we so choose. The concern is thus that a child's welfare is anchored on nothing more secure than individual consent.

Cahill herself rejects this interpretation of her argument, but it is important to see the problems with this line of reasoning because other opponents of assisted reproduction will find it attractive. In this interpretation, attention to "natural [biological] kinship bonds" reveals that biological relation offers children greater moral protection from abandonment than the parental bonds to which individuals freely consent in undertaking assisted reproduction with donor gametes.[20] The obvious question is, Does it? While it may be true that biological relation will often, in Cahill's words, "undergird and enhance" the interpersonal relation between parent and child, this biological relation is not necessary to the development of an intense, ongoing social relationship, nor does the existence of biological relation ensure a social commitment to care.

In this interpretation, Cahill's comment that biological relation will often "undergird and enhance" the social relation between a parent and child is understood to point to a significant problem with my view of parenthood. In this view, to define parenthood primarily in social terms is somehow to diminish the responsibilities for which we hold parents accountable. Where Kass suggests that genetic connection grounds a privileged parental claim, this view suggests that genetic connection grounds more substantial moral obligations. Both positions are mistaken. The latter one is mistaken because, although defining the commitment to care as the hallmark of responsible parenthood does indeed place considerable emphasis on choice, it does not make the responsibilities of parenthood "entirely contingent on choice." To be sure, had the couple chosen differently, the child would not exist. Yet once they have committed themselves to care for and nurture a child, their obligations cannot be simply willed out of existence.

This is why I think Cahill's argument is mistaken, whether it is interpreted as a natural law argument or as a strictly consequentialist one. It is just not true to say that to affirm surrogacy and other forms of assisted reproduction that involve the use of donor gametes is "to affirm that the only morally binding relationships are the ones to which persons freely consent."[21] To decide to bring a child into existence through donor insemination is to choose commitment and thus to consent freely to a morally binding relationship. There is thus a sense in which obligation is contingent on the consent. It does not follow, however, that the relationship ceases to be binding morally if the parents withdraw their consent. The father of a child produced through donor insemination is every bit as obligated to care for the child he has created as the father of the child conceived through intercourse. And we ought to make the same judgment about a parent who ignores his obligation, whether the child was created through assisted reproduction or not.

Thus it seems to me that we should reject Cahill's claim that creating a child with the intention of separating genetic and social parenthood is morally unacceptable. Doing so threatens neither the core of parenthood nor the stringency of parental obligations. Parental responsibilities are, in a sense, inalienable, but it is not genetic connection that makes them so; rather, it is the intense, person-specific nature of the interpersonal bonds that constitute the parental relation that makes parental responsibility largely nontransferable. So Cahill's objection to the intentional separation of genetic and social parenthood is unfounded. Are there other reasons for believing donor insemination may be wrong?

I think there are reasons for concern about donor insemination, but unlike those we examined in the works of Kass and Cahill, these reasons are distinct from a consideration of whether the mere separation of genetic and social parenthood is itself morally problematic: these reasons are distinct from any claims about the intrinsic or ontological significance of separating genetic and social parenthood. Instead, we must consider what the effects of intentionally separating genetic and social parenthood are on responsible parenthood. We must ask whether there is anything about creating a child who will not be cared for by his/her biological parents that stands as a significant obstacle to the activities of nurturing that child or that frustrates the goal of that care, namely, the growth and well-being of the child. Notice that to ask this question is not to ask, as some insist we must, whether donor insemination is undertaken for the sake of the child, rather than for the sake of the couple.[22] It seems to me that this contrast is largely meaningless and is not, in any event, one that would distinguish donor insemination from any other form of reproduction. To ask this question, however, is to draw attention to the fact that it is responsible parenthood that we want to promote, and deciding responsibly about parenthood involves asking whether one is capable of meeting the demands of parenting and whether one can reasonably expect the child to flourish in one's care. Just as we should expect a couple who are contemplating parenthood, but who do not require assisted reproduction, to consider whether they can properly care for a child at that particular point in time and under some particular set of circumstances, so we should expect a couple considering donor insemination to consider whether they can properly care for a child conceived in this particular way. So is there something about conceiving a child through donor insemination that poses a threat to that child's future well-being?

I want to focus on two such dangers that donor insemination poses for responsible parenthood. The first arises from the secrecy that now typically surrounds donor insemination. The second emerges from the asymmetry that donor insemination creates between the mother of the donor child, who is both the biological and the social mother, and the father of the child, who is the social but not the biological father. The first obstacle is a function of the current practice of donor insemination, and I will argue that practice can and should be changed. The second obstacle is less tractable, but it is not, I will argue, an insuperable barrier to responsible parenthood.

The Problem of Secrecy

One of the most striking features of donor insemination as it is currently practiced is the secrecy that surrounds it. Although the Office of Technology Assessment estimates that approximately 30,000 children are born every year of donor insemination in the United States, very little is known about these children, their parents, or the donors. There are a number of reasons for this lack of information. Because no formal process exists for screening prospective donor parents such as exists with adoption and because the husband of the child's mother is typically listed as the child's father on the birth certificate there is little public information available even about general trends associated with donor insemination; specific information is even harder to obtain. According to the OTA, only about half of the physicians doing donor inseminations keep records sufficiently specific to permit them to identify a particular donor for a particular pregnancy, and a majority would not release recorded information to anyone, even if all identifying information were removed.[23]

The fact that so little public information is available on donor insemination, however, does not necessarily mean that donor insemination is typically undertaken in secret. There is a difference between privacy and secrecy, and physicians may protect the confidentiality of the physician-patient relationship as indeed they may protect the privacy of sperm donors by assuring anonymity without counseling or sanctioning secrecy.[24] Nevertheless, it appears that most physicians counsel prospective donor parents to keep the truth about donor insemination not simply private but secret, that is, hidden from immediate family and the child. The view of the Royal College of Obstetricians and Gynecologists appears to be the norm. "Unless you [the parents] decide to tell the child," they write, "there is no reason for him (or her) ever to know that he (or she) was conceived by AID."[25] The clear implication is that if there is no reason to know, there is no reason for the couple to decide to tell the child. Add to this the fact that the few studies that have queried prospective donor parents have found that the majority either decided not to tell the child the truth about his or her conception or were undecided about whether to tell the truth as they actually began donor insemination, and we can safely conclude that donor insemination is most frequently undertaken in secrecy and that the lack of detailed record-keeping is often a form of collusion in the maintenance of the secret.[26] My experience certainly bears this out. When donor insemination was offered to my wife and me as a possible form of treatment, we were advised by the head of the donor program not to tell the child because the child did not need to know. Can such secrecy be justified morally?

My own view is that it cannot. Indeed, I believe that the secrecy in which donor insemination is now typically undertaken is a serious obstacle to responsible parenthood and thus a reason to oppose this form of assisted reproduction in many cases. To keep the truth about a child's conception hidden from him is, at least in theory if not always in practice, to plant at the heart of the parent-child relationship the seed of its undoing and the potential for serious psychological and emotional harm to the child.

That secrecy cannot be justified in relation to donor insemination can be seen by examining the reasons for and against maintaining the secrecy and exploring the likely consequences of keeping this information hidden. As Ken Daniels has pointed out, a variety of explanations have been offered to account for the secrecy surrounding donor insemination.[27] Three of the suggested explanations appear to be plausible reasons to which parents might appeal to justify secrecy. First, it might be argued that the truth should be concealed to protect the child from any stigma or disapprobation that is associated with donor insemination. Since donor insemination is not particularly common, and since donor insemination is still controversial, to tell the child that he or she was conceived through DI is to put the child at risk of feeling, or being treated as, marginal. So one reason is to protect the child.

A second reason is to protect the donor. George Annas has suggested that this is the primary reason donor insemination is conducted in secret.[28] Because so few states have, until recently, addressed the issue surrounding the legal rights and responsibilities of parenthood in DI cases, secrecy protected the donor from liability for child support for any children produced through DI or from claims of inheritance from such offspring. Since the legal situation was uncertain, secrecy protected the donor from legal responsibility and thus ensured a reliable pool of donors, who might otherwise refuse to participate. Physicians who counsel secrecy may thus be understood as acting to protect the anonymity of donors in order to ensure a continued supply of sperm, and parents who embrace secrecy may be understood as acting to protect the donor in order to protect themselves from an unwelcome and unexpected assertion of parental rights on the part of the donor as biological father.

If the first argument for secrecy is to protect the child and the second is to protect the donor, the third is to protect the infertile husband. In their study of donor insemination, for example, Baran and Pannor found that many of the infertile men who consented to donor insemination to overcome childlessness did so "because it would permit them to appear fertile in the eyes of the outside world."[29] Indeed, Baran and Pannor suggest that one of the reasons donor insemination may be so popular as a form of treatment for male infertility is that it offers an infertile man the hope that he may feel fertile if he appears fertile. Secrecy, however, is necessary to protect the appearance of fertility, and so secrecy protects an infertile husband by allowing him to avoid the pain and embarrassment of public recognition of his inability to father a child. Baran and Pannor are not alone in suggesting this explanation. Drawing on in-depth interviews with sixty couples who are parents of DI children, Snowden also concluded that the main reason for secrecy was to protect an infertile husband from public disclosure of his problem.[30]

What reasons weigh against secrecy? The primary reason is that to hide the truth about a child's conception from him is to build the parent-child relationship on a foundation of deception. I have, of course, already rejected the claim that the parent-child bond requires a biological base, but this is not to say that we may put a fiction in its place. Indeed, to reject the necessity of biological connection to relational bonds is to reject the necessity of lying about biological connection to ensure those bonds. Notice that in rejecting secrecy here I am not saying that a child has a right to know his or her biological parents; this is a stronger and more controversial claim.[31] Nor am I saying that a parent-child bond depends upon complete or total honesty. Rather, I am suggesting that there must not be deception at the core of the parent-child relationship. Such a relationship depends on truth telling, and it creates expectations of truthfulness that will be violated when a child is misled about such a basic matter as the identity of the biological father. At the very least, not telling the child the truth about donor insemination will be deceptive. Even if the child never asks directly about his origins, even if the parents do not have to lie about the conception, they will be intentionally deceiving the child, who will reasonably assume that he is the biological offspring of his parents.

Unfortunately, the deception is unlikely to end with merely withholding the truth. As Sisela Bok has noted, lies are particularly corrosive and contagious within families. "The need to shore up lies, [to] keep them in good repair," she writes, "the anxieties relating to possible discovery, the entanglements and threats to integrity—are greatest in a close relationship where it is rare that one lie will suffice."[32] The truth of what Bok says here is even more striking when we extend her reasoning to cover, not one isolated incident of lying in a close relationship, but a whole relationship built on a lie. Indeed, the notion of "living a lie" seems particularly apt to capture a father's relation to a donor child from whom he has kept the truth. The pattern of deceit that such a life involves is simply incompatible with the commitments that responsible parenthood entails.

Deceit is incompatible with responsible parenthood, not simply in theory but in practice as well. The effort to "live a lie" will be accompanied by a sense of shame and guilt that will do nothing to foster the parent-child relationship. On the contrary, the anxiety that comes from persistent evasiveness and from the constant fear of disclosure will be a significant barrier between parent and child. Where trust should be paramount, we can expect fear and suspicion: the father's fear of being discovered, the child's suspicion that all is not what it seems. This is precisely what Baran and Pannor found in their study of seventy donor insemination families and nineteen donor offspring, and the picture they draw of the consequences of keeping donor insemination secret is so disturbing, it is worth looking briefly at their findings.

According to Baran and Pannor, the destructive dynamic of secrecy is readily discerned. When donor insemination is used to circumvent male infertility, secrecy is attractive because it allows an infertile male to hide his problem from everyone, save his spouse. Unfortunately, to mask a problem is not to resolve it, and secrecy only serves to delay an acknowledgment of the emotional and psychological effects of sterility. Infertile individuals need to mourn and grieve the children they will not produce, they need to resolve any feelings of inadequacies that sterility may engender, and secrecy is an obstacle to meeting both needs. The upshot of undertaking donor insemination without resolving these difficulties, however, is that the relationship of the parents to each other and to any children they may raise together is fundamentally altered. The man's spouse knows the truth about his inadequacy and becomes more powerful; the child is a constant reminder of that inadequacy and may be treated accordingly.

Baran and Pannor summarize their findings as follows:

> For most of the men we interviewed, the choice of donor insemination had been an acute response to the pain they were experiencing. They never permitted themselves the time and opportunity to explore their feelings about the devastating ego blow. They prevented themselves from becoming comfortable with and accepting of their handicap. Instead, they cast the handicap in concrete, and their feelings of inadequacy were continuously reinforced by visual proof: their donor offspring.
>
> With this enormous deficit in place, the relationship between the husband and wife had to be realigned. The husband became weaker and more passive; the wife became stronger and more powerful. The wife was the real mother of the children, and this message, although never spoken, was clearly given to the husband in many ways. The husband could be devoted and caring toward the children, while at the same time recognizing the difference between his parental role and his wife's.[33]

Moreover, according to Baran and Pannor, the children in donor insemination families are generally aware of the difference in roles played by their parents and are often suspicious that something is not right with their family. Further, however hard the parents work at maintaining the secret, disclosure is only an angry word away. Many children will thus learn the truth ultimately in any event, often under the worst possible circumstances. This was true of the donor children Baran and Pannor interviewed, almost all of whom "had learned the truth of their origins in a punitive manner, when their parents' relationship began to disintegrate."[34] It will not be surprising to learn that discovery of the truth under these circumstances was deeply traumatic. Baran and Pannor concluded that, for all the parties involved, secrecy is destructive. It is destructive of the parents' relationship to one another because it reinforces a sense of failure that will interfere with truly equal and cooperative parenting. It is destructive of the parents' relationship to a child because it is grounded on an unstable foundation. When secrecy is the norm, a donor child may become an unwelcome reminder of unresolved failure or a potential weapon in a power struggle between the parents or both.

In my terminology, secrecy is a serious obstacle to responsible parenting. If I am right that responsible parenting should be both the goal we seek to promote and the standard by which we judge assisted reproduction, then at the very least we should be skeptical about the legitimacy of donor insemination as it is currently practiced. When we further consider the reasons given for secrecy in light of the reasons given against it, we cannot but conclude that donor insemination undertaken in secret is morally unacceptable. Recall the reasons for maintaining secrecy. The first was that secrecy protects the child from harm. Given the impact that secrecy is likely to have on the parent-child relationship, we may well ask whether secrecy causes more harm that it could possibly prevent. Moreover, even if it were the case that harm came to the child as the result of being conceived in a way not fully accepted by everyone in our society, it does not follow that donor insemination should then be undertakn in secret. Rather than hide the truth, the appropriate response would be to combat the fear and prejudice that causes donor insemination to be stigmatized or to avoid donor insemination altogether in order to avoid possible harm.

The second and third reasons to maintain secrecy fare no better. As we have seen, secrecy to hide the embarrassment of infertility hides, too, the pain and suffering that accompany it. Secrecy thus protects the infertile from embarrassment, but at a very high price. When pain and anger cannot be acknowledged, they cannot be resolved either. Behind the mask of apparent fertility, there is likely to be the clenched jaw of resentment. So secrecy to protect an infertile man from embarrassment appears problematic even as a measure to protect a husband from harm. Is protection of the donor any more compelling a reason to keep donor insemination a secret?

In one sense, of course, this question supervenes upon the question of whether donor insemination, with or without secrecy, is morally acceptable. If the concern in protecting donors is to ensure a pool of available donors in order to maintain the practice of donor insemination, then we first need to know whether the practice is worth saving. Yet even if we reach the conclusion, as I have, that donor insemination in general is morally acceptable, it does not follow that secrecy is justified to maintain the practice or even that it is necessary. I have already suggested implicitly why I think truthfulness is not incompatible with donor anonymity, at least for a considerable period of time. If we draw a distinction between secrecy and privacy, then it makes sense to affirm openness while nevertheless guarding privacy and anonymity, constrained only by concern for the well-being of the child.

The Problem of Asymmetry

We began our discussion of secrecy in donor insemination in response to the question of whether there is anything about conceiving a child through DI that stands as an obstacle to discharging the core commitments of responsible parenthood. I suggested that although secrecy is not a constitutive feature of donor insemination, it is a pervasive part of current DI practice and is in fact a barrier to the development of a healthy parent-child relationship. I now consider an aspect of donor insemination that is a constitutive feature of the practice and that many think is an obstacle to responsible parenthood, namely, the asymmetry between the mother's relation to the child and the father's. The difference between the two relations is clear: the mother is both a biological and social parent to the child, whereas the father is only a social parent. Will this difference impede responsible parenting?

I have already suggested that the mere absence of genetic connection does not bar the development of a caring nurturing relationship of a social parent to a child. The evidence from adoption is clear on this point. It is important to notice, however, that donor insemination is here quite different from adoption. In the case of adoption, a couple is in the same position vis-à-vis the child: neither is a biological parent, both are social parents. With donor insemination, this is not the case. The mother is the biological parent, and the father is not. We have seen from the study undertaken by Baran and Pannor that when this discrepancy in relation is kept secret, it easily contributes to a power struggle between the parents that has a deleterious effect on the father's relation to the child. At the very least, then, donor insemination is different from adoption in that we can expect the absence of a genetic relation to have greater significance in donor insemination than in adoption. Even if the asymmetry is not kept secret, it may contribute to stress in the marriage that would not exist in the case of adoption. For there is a difference between the mother's relation to the child and the father's that is ineradicable; it can be overcome but it cannot be eliminated.

Overcoming this difference, however, may prove extremely difficult.

When the child is young, there will be the inevitable speculation by others about whom the child resembles. For the father this is likely to be painful and to frustrate rather than further the parent-child bond. If the child develops in a way or with interests unlike the father, or if the child is particularly close to the mother, the father may feel left out. If the child is told about the conception, he is likely at some point to wield this information like a blunt instrument to inflict pain. He may shout in anger that he hates his mother, but it is only to his father that he will say that he is not his real parent. So the absence of genetic relation is likely to be painful and isolating, and this is a pain and isolation that the mother cannot fully share.

This last point about the inability to fully share the experience of parenting is important because it may help us to understand one fairly common objection to donor insemination, namely, that it is a form of marital infidelity. This claim may appear puzzling at first. Donor insemination need not involve sexual contact between the woman and the donor, and it will usually be undertaken with the full knowledge and consent of the partners in a marriage, who may undertake donor insemination out of a commitment to their marriage.[35] To some critics, however, these basic facts are irrelevant; DI is a form of infidelity by definition. James Burtchaell, for example, insists that DI is adultery, whatever the facts. Yet even a cursory examination of his reasoning shows how tendentious this view is. "If intercourse is sex even without impregnation," Burtchaell writes, "then impregnation even without intercourse must also be sex."[36] Thus does assertion defeat argument.

Nevertheless, although the claim that donor insemination involves sexual infidelity is unfounded, we must not dismiss the general concern here too quickly. The general objection has been raised, for example, in the Vatican *Instruction* on assisted reproduction: "The fidelity of the spouses in the unity of marriage involves reciprocal respect of their right to become a father and a mother only through each other."[37] Since donor insemination does not protect this right, it is a form of adultery and therefore is wrong. How does donor insemination involve infidelity? What does the Vatican have in mind in making this charge? The answer is revealed in the fact that the Vatican document links fidelity and *unity*. "Fidelity of the spouses *in the unity of marriage*" is the norm offered by the Vatican. "Heterologous artificial fertilization," we read, "is contrary to the unity of marriage. . . ." Or again: "Recourse to the gametes of a third person in order to have sperm or ovum available constitutes a violation of the reciprocal commitment of the spouses and a grave lack in regard to that essential property of marriage which is its unity."[38] To claim that donor insemination is a form of adultery because it violates marital unity is much more plausible than to say the DI violates either sexual or emotional fidelity. Conceiving a child through donor insemination may introduce a series of important life experiences into a marriage that cannot be fully shared, however committed a couple is to one another. This lack of mutuality may interfere with the couple's ability to care for and to love the child that is created.

The question, of course, is whether the disunity that donor insemination may introduce into a relationship is an overwhelming obstacle to responsible parenthood. The answer, it seems to me, is that it is not. To be sure, we must not dismiss this concern too quickly. The potential for significant conflict exists, and this conflict could lead to serious harm to the child. Yet we must also acknowledge that the potential for conflict or disunity exists whenever a child is created, and the circumstances that increase the potential for conflict in this instance are not so different from those in other cases that we currently accept. So-called blended families in which children are raised by a biological parent and a nonbiological parent experience many of the same difficulties raised by donor insemination. Nevertheless, in the case of blended families we believe that a committed relation based on honesty, trust, and respect can overcome the difficulties that everyone acknowledges. The same can be said of donor insemination. No one should be deceived about the difficulties that may arise when parenthood is pursued in this way, but neither should the pitfalls be exaggerated.

In asking what impact the secrecy or the asymmetry of donor insemination may have on the parent-child relationship or on the relationship of a couple to one another, we are raising questions about the possible obstacles posed for responsible parenthood by donor insemination. We can ask questions of this sort from two vantage points: from the parent's perspective or from that of the child. Thus far we have focused primarily on the parent's perspective. I have suggested that the secrecy that surrounds DI and the asymmetry that will always accompany it can interfere with the parent's ability to establish the sort of caring relationship with the child that is the heart of responsible parenthood. Where this is the case—almost always with secrecy, sometimes with asymmetry—donor insemination is a morally impermissible way to pursue parenthood. What if we now ask about the obstacles to the goals of responsible parenting from the child's vantage point? Is there something about being conceived in this way that is a barrier to human flourishing, irrespective of the impact of the conception on the parent's ability to care for the child?

Presumably, such a concern stands behind the Vatican's claim that donor insemination is wrong, not only because it is a form of infidelity, but because it violates a child's right to be born to, and brought up within, a heterosexual marriage. In other words, it might be argued that however lovingly cared for a child may be, he has lost something irreplaceable in being conceived through DI. This appears to be the Vatican view. "Heterologous artificial fertilization," we read, "violates the rights of the child; it deprives him of his filial relationship with his parental origins."[39] We have already discussed the conceptual oddity of claiming that an individual's rights have been violated by being conceived in a certain way.

Nevertheless, the Vatican concern here can be expressed without appeal to the notion of rights and is relatively clear.

Leon Kass has made essentially the same claim, only more directly and in the language of respect. According to Kass, donor insemination and other forms of assisted reproduction that use donor gametes fail to respect what it means to be human. To pursue parenthood in these ways is to fail to respect the full humanity of the child so created because "to be human means not only to have human form and powers; it means also to have a human context and to be humanly connected."[40] To be conceived through donor insemination is thus to be robbed of the full measure of one's humanity because one is stripped of the connection of biological kinship. To recall the Vatican language, one is deprived of filial relationship by being cut loose from parental origins. The point for both the Vatican and for Kass appears to be that a person so conceived is not whole.

If we attend to this line of argument more carefully, however, we can see that however deontological the cast of the argument, its real form is consequentialist. When the Vatican says that this sort of conception is incompatible with the respect the fetus deserves as a person from the moment of conception and when Kass says that to be bound up with biological ancestors is part of what it means to be human, neither is suggesting that the child who is conceived through donor insemination is not fully deserving of respect or somehow not fully human. Rather, the concern is that there will be deleterious consequences to the child of being conceived in this way. In the Vatican *Instruction* we read, "It is through the secure and recognized relationship to his own [biological] parents that the child can discover his own identity and achieve his own proper human development," and in Kass we find, "Clarity about your origins is crucial for self-identity, itself important for self-respect."[41] In other words, the real objection to donor insemination at this point is that it does not matter how loving, caring, and nurturing the parents of a donor child are; such a child is unlikely to flourish because he will not have what is necessary for the development of a stable sense of self-identity, namely, relation with or knowledge about both biological parents.

Is there evidence to support this claim? The unequivocal answer is that there is not. In his 1987 review of the literature on donor insemination, Jarrett Richardson discovered that only 430 children produced through donor insemination have been directly studied and these children only through the very first years of life. His assessment of the literature is clear: "These studies do not provide significant enlightenment on the questions of paternal acceptance of the child in the long term or on the long-term psychological integrity of an AID child."[42] Moreover, the slightly more numerous studies that have focused on the impact of donor insemination on couples rather than on their children are not helpful either. In most of these cases, the children do not know about their origins, and thus we fail to get even indirect evidence about the likely impact of donor insemination on self-identity from knowledge about the overall stability or lack of stability of the family unit.[43]

In fact, the only evidence to support the claim that donor insemination will harm the development of self-identity in a donor child appears to be based on the view, first, that the lack of information about genetic parents is harmful to adopted children and, second, that donor children will develop like adopted children. Both of these convictions are problematic. The first presupposes that there is an identifiable condition generally referred to in the literature on adoption as "genealogical bewilderment." According to this theory, the lack of knowledge or the limited knowledge that an adopted child has about his biological parents results in a state of confusion that undermines his security and identity.[44] The second conviction presupposes that because a donor child has limited or no knowledge about his biological father, he will respond in the same confused way as the adopted child who knows little or nothing about either parent.

The problem with these assumptions is that they are open to serious doubt. While it is true that adopted children sometimes search for their biological parents—the actual percentage that do is hotly debated—and while adopted children will sometimes have a very fragile sense of identity, it is an open question whether searching for one's biological parents is evidence of maladjustment or whether a fragile ego is a result of genealogical bewilderment. Michael Humphrey has argued, for example, that the empirical evidence does not support the claim that lack of information about genetic ancestors is a significant contributor to maladjustment. In adoptive families where the parent-child relationship is sufficient to meet the emotional needs of the child, information about biological parents is not a prerequisite for a stable sense of self or for mental health generally.[45] Indeed, we can see the difficulty of establishing the opposite view.[46] In cases where maladjustment is associated with a lack of identity or with a compulsion to search for biological parents we will need to ask whether the maladjustment, based, say, on a lack of acceptance by the adoptive parents, caused the insecurity about identity or whether this insecurity, based on the lack of genealogical information, caused the maladjustment. How we will answer this question is unclear. Further, even if we can be certain that the absence of information about biological parents affects adopted children adversely, how can we be sure the same adverse effects will appear in donor children? Given that adopted children often report feeling abandoned by their biological parents and given that that feeling will frequently be an obstacle to the development of a healthy sense of self-esteem, can we assume a similar psychological dynamic in donor insemination where the notion of abandonment makes no sense?

Yet even if we could document genealogical bewilderment as an obstacle to proper self-development in a child, and even if we could demonstrate that the effects of genealogical bewilderment will be the same in donor insemination as in adoption, the most we could conclude is that information about donors should be accessible to the children if they request it. In other words, even if Kass or the Vatican is correct that a child conceived through donor insemination is unlikely to flourish without knowledge of his biological father, it does not follow that donor insemination is morally wrong. The most that could be said to follow here is that donor insemination should be structured in such a way that donor children can obtain information about their biological fathers.

In one sense, of course, the recommendation that donor children should have access to information about their biological fathers is simply an extension of the view that donor insemination should not be undertaken in secret. I agree with the conclusions reached by Baran and Pannor. Donor insemination must not be a darkly hidden secret. Donor children should be told of their origins, and this means more than identifying a biological father as a mysterious ejaculator. In Baran and Pannor's words, the "donor father is a real person, not a teaspoonful of sperm," and the donor child should be able to know the identity of the real person at an appropriate age, if he so chooses.[47]

If donor insemination were to become not only not secret but open, then any remaining force to the objection that separating genetic and social parenthood is an obstacle to the proper emotional development of the child is dissipated. For even if knowledge of biological ancestry is central to self-respect, the child would have access to this information, if needed. So I conclude that the concerns raised by the Vatican and by Leon Kass about the respect owed to the donor child are not sufficient to justify wholesale opposition to donor insemination. At best they argue against a process of donor insemination that is closed and secretive.

If we step back at this point and consider what conclusions we should draw about the use of donor gametes now that we have completed our review of the major objections to donor insemination, several things stand out. First, a strong case can be made for defining parenthood primarily in relational terms. We saw that when, as in the case of Kimberly Mays, we are forced to choose between genetic connection and social/emotional connection, we appropriately opt for social relation.[48] To place value in this way on the rearing component of parenthood, however, is to begin to identify criteria by which we can assess forms of assisted reproduction. Rearing a child is a social practice that requires certain virtues and that has standards of success integral to the practice. The development of an intense, nurturing relationship is central to the practice of rearing a child, and virtues such as patience, honesty, and compassion are central to the development of a loving and caring relationship. The practice itself, of course, aims to foster the growth and development of a person from infancy to adulthood in a way that promotes human flourishing. So we can meaningfully speak about standards of responsible parenthood in relation to both the ultimate goals of the practice of parenting and the virtues necessary to realize these goals.[49]

Viewing donor insemination in relation to these standards, our assessment can only be mixed. As it is currently practiced, in secret and in many cases without any possibility of obtaining information about the donor, DI will often fail to meet the standards of responsible parenthood. Secrecy can be a profound obstacle to the development of a loving and healthy parent-child relationship. Undertaken in secret, donor insemination will eclipse one of the central virtues of responsible parenthood, namely, honesty. Even where donor insemination is openly acknowledged, however, we have seen that the separation of genetic and social parenthood and the asymmetry it entails introduce burdens that are significantly different from and greater than those associated with traditional parenting. We should not deceive ourselves into thinking that everyone who considers undertaking DI will be capable of responsibly meeting these additional burdens.

Nevertheless, given the standard of responsible parenthood, we cannot categorically reject donor insemination as morally wrong. If we value the rearing function of parenthood more highly than the genetic relation of biological parenthood, and if we assess forms of pursuing parenthood in relation to the standards of responsible parenthood so conceived, we will conclude that donor insemination can be a perfectly acceptable form of assisted reproduction. We have seen that there is nothing about intentionally creating a child who will be raised by her biological mother and the mother's spouse that is inherently incompatible with responsible parenthood, considered either from the parents' or from the child's point of view.

Implications for IVF with Egg Donation

The other conclusion that emerges at this point is that if we do not preemptively and arbitrarily rule out the use of third-party gametes, then we will need to ask whether the arguments that support the qualified endorsement of donor insemination given above also serve to justify *in vitro* fertilization with donor eggs. I did not consider the use of IVF with donor eggs in my previous discussion of IVF because this particular form of assisted reproduction is best considered together with donor insemination. Although the comparison to donor insemination is most frequently found in discussions of surrogate motherhood, in fact the real equivalent to donor insemination in the treatment of female infertility is IVF with donor eggs. For just as donor insemination provides the missing gametes to a couple in the case of male infertility, so does IVF with egg donation provide the gametes to a couple in the case of female infertility. To be sure, there are differences between the use of donor sperm via artificial insemination and the use of donor eggs via IVF followed by implantation. Nevertheless, there are striking similarities that lead us to ask, Does the argument for donor insemination set out above also support IVF with donor eggs?

The answer is that it does. If we accept IVF in general—as I argued we should in chapter 2—and if we conditionally accept artificial insemination with donor sperm—as I have just argued we should—it follows that we should also accept the use of IVF with donor eggs. In one crucial respect the two forms of assisted reproduction are identical: both use donor gametes in order to overcome infertility. So both confront the difficulties associated with asymmetry and, if the asymmetry is not acknowledged, with secrecy. Yet we have seen in the case of DI that neither asymmetry nor secrecy necessarily raises insurmountable obstacles to responsible parenting. Secrecy may be avoided and the potential strains of asymmetry may be mediated by an honest, loving, and straightforward acknowledgment of the differences between families created through the use of donor gametes and those created "naturally."

In fact, we can now see that, in relation to one of the two ways in which IVF with egg donation differs significantly from DI, it is less problematic. The difference arises from the fact that the woman who receives the donated egg is not simply the social parent of the child, but the gestational parent as well. Because the woman who receives the donation gestates the resulting embryo, there exists a biological relationship between her child and herself that does not exist between a donor insemination child and her social father.[50] Thus, although there is still an asymmetry between the child's mother and father, it is not nearly so pronounced here as with donor insemination. The social mother will have nurtured the child physically/biologically for nine months, and although the child will not have received her basic chromosomal structure from her mother, the interaction between the developing fetus and the gestating mother will significantly affect the phenotypic expression of the child's genotype. Add to this the fact that a mother who has carried a child to term and quite probably nursed that child is unlikely to feel inadequate, or to have her identity threatened by her "infertility," and we can see that IVF with egg donation may well be less complicated emotionally and less challenging to responsible parenting than is donor insemination. Far from being a constant reminder of perceived failure and inadequacy, the child produced through egg donation will likely be an ever-present affirmation of what is arguably the most significant accomplishment of human reproduction, namely, the power of gestation. In other words, where donor insemination can only be misleadingly labeled a treatment for male infertility, IVF with egg donation may legitimately be called a treatment for female infertility. While donor insemination does not allow a man to conceive a child that is genetically his offspring and while it does not allow him with his partner to have a child who is, to borrow Kass's words again, "flesh of their flesh," the same is not true for IVF with donor eggs. At the very least, there is a real sense in which the child is "flesh of their flesh," and, as I pointed out, there will be some genetic impact as well. So IVF with donor eggs overcomes female infertility in a way that donor insemination does not overcome male infertility. In precisely those ways, IVF with donor eggs will be less morally problematic than donor insemination.[51]

Can the same thing be said about surrogate motherhood, the other form of assisted reproduction that has been compared to donor insemination? It is to this question that I turn in the next chapter.

5

Parenting for Profit

Problems with Surrogate Motherhood

Surrogate motherhood is frequently compared to artificial insemination with donor sperm. Indeed, supporters of surrogacy would like nothing better than to see public policy on donor insemination become the accepted paradigm for handling surrogate motherhood. Surrogacy is repeatedly compared to donor insemination in the literature on surrogate motherhood, and the comparison is drawn precisely to suggest that DI should be the paradigm for surrogacy. Since states recognize and facilitate DI, it is argued, they should recognize and facilitate surrogate motherhood. Unfortunately, the exact nature of the connection between surrogacy and donor insemination is rarely explored. Surrogacy is said to be the "converse" of donor insemination,[1] its "reverse,"[2] its "flipside,"[3] and its "mirror" image,[4] and these comparisons are invoked as if it followed from the fact that surrogacy is, say, the mirror image of donor insemination that surrogacy should be treated morally and legally as we treat donor insemination.

Does it follow? Should we reach the same moral conclusions about surrogate motherhood? The answer is no, at least where commercial surrogacy is concerned. Acknowledging the similarities between surrogate motherhood and donor insemination should not obscure their differences, and these differences are significant. Let us begin, then, by attending to the similarities and differences.

Comparing Surrogacy and Donor Insemination: Equal Protection Arguments for Surrogacy

Consider, first, the legal battle over surrogacy. Court cases have frequently turned on the question of whether surrogate motherhood is like or unlike donor insemination. The Kentucky Supreme Court held that payment to a surrogate did not violate Kentucky statutes against baby selling because the man who contracts with the surrogate is the biological father and because surrogacy does not differ essentially from the legally sanctioned activity of donor insemination. As the court put it, surrogate motherhood "is not biologically different from the reverse situation where the husband is infertile and the wife conceives by artificial insemination."[5] If the one is legally permitted, the court reasoned, so should be the other.

Similarly, in the famous Baby M case, the Superior Court of New Jersey held that a constitutionally protected right exists to procreate through surrogate parenting agreements. Again, justification for this position relied on an explicit comparison to donor insemination agreements. The court wrote: "Currently, males may sell their sperm. The 'surrogate father' sperm donor is legally recognized in all states. The surrogate mother is not. If a man may offer the means for procreation then a woman must equally be allowed to do so."[6] Thus, the New Jersey Superior Court also held that surrogate contracts were legally valid, in part because the contracts are similar to donor insemination arrangements. By contrast, the New Jersey Supreme Court rejected the comparison between surrogate motherhood and donor insemination and ruled that the surrogate mother contract was not only unenforceable, but void and possibly criminal.

Clearly, the comparison to donor insemination is important to the legal controversy over surrogate motherhood. Where the similarity to donor insemination is stressed, we can expect to see legal rulings in favor of surrogacy. Where the dissimilarity is highlighted, surrogacy will be looked on less favorably.

Although I do not wish to undertake an extensive review of the legal issues surrounding surrogacy, it is worth pausing briefly to consider why, legally, so much appears to turn on the question of whether surrogacy is like donor insemination. The reason is nicely illustrated by the case of Baby M. The basic facts of this case are undisputed and well known. In February 1985, William Stern signed a surrogate parenting contract with Mary Beth and Richard Whitehead, which provided that Mary Beth Whitehead would, for a fee, be inseminated with William Stern's sperm, carry any child so conceived to term, surrender the child to Mr. Stern at birth, and relinquish at that time any parental rights to the child. On March 27, 1986, Baby M, the child of Mary Beth Whitehead and William Stern, was born. Mary Beth Whitehead then refused to abide by the terms of the contract (i.e., she refused to turn over Baby M or to relinquish parental rights and responsibilities), and William Stern filed suit to have the surrogate contract enforced. On January 5, 1987, the highly publicized case of Baby M went to trial.

From the start of the trial, one of the central questions was whether William Stern had a constitutionally protected right to procreate through the use of a surrogate mother contract. It was in relation to this question that the comparison to donor insemination became important. William Stern argued that to invalidate the surrogacy contract would be to deny him equal protection under the law as guaranteed by the Fourteenth Amendment. The logic of equal protection claims explains why the comparison to donor insemination was crucial. To establish a violation of the equal protection clause, one must demonstrate that a particular group has been disadvantaged by the law as compared to a similarly situated group.[7] In this case, William Stern claimed that he was in the same position as a woman who seeks DI to overcome her husband's infertility. In both cases, a person with an infertile spouse seeks to procreate with a third party who relinquishes all parental rights and responsibilities. So long as donor insemination is legal, Stern reasoned, surrogate mother contracts must be legally protected or the state will unfairly favor couples with male infertility over couples with female infertility.

The New Jersey Superior Court accepted this argument because it accepted the comparison between surrogacy and donor insemination. "Classifications of persons to be sustained for equal protection purposes," Judge Sorkow wrote, "'must be reasonable, not arbitrary and must rest upon some ground of difference having a fair and substantial relation to the object of the legislation so that all persons similarly circumstanced shall be treated alike.'"[8] Since Judge Sorkow found no reasonable difference between surrogacy and donor insemination, he concluded that to disallow surrogacy contracts would deny equal protection to "the childless couple, the surrogate, whether male or female, and the unborn child." We can certainly see how Judge Sorkow came to this conclusion. To be sure, the formal similarities are striking. Both donor insemination and surrogate motherhood, for example, involve preconception termination of parental rights. Indeed, the procedures can be described in identical terms, as a form of assisted reproduction in which artificial insemination is used to produce a child who is genetically related to at least one partner in an infertile couple. There are thus indisputable similarities.

Yet if we look more closely at the analogy, we can also see very good reasons to question both the appeal to the equal protection clause and the comparison of surrogacy to donor insemination, despite the formal resemblance. Capron and Radin have pointed out, for example, that even on a formal level the comparison fails to ground an equal protection claim because the laws adopted to facilitate donor insemination can be applied in the context of surrogacy. In fact, although it is rarely framed in this way, surrogacy involves donor insemination. Describing the man who initiates the contract as something other than a "donor" does not change the fact that a woman consents to being artificially inseminated with the sperm of someone other than her husband. That, of course, is precisely what happens in the case of donor insemination, and state laws that cover this form of procreation apply equally to surrogate parenting arrangements. That state laws governing donor insemination do apply in the context of surrogacy is demonstrated by the fact that the husbands of surrogates typically sign a statement of nonconsent to their wives' insemination. If such a form is not signed, the husband of the surrogate will be presumed to be the legal father of the child under donor insemination laws. So, even granting the similarities between donor insemination and surrogacy, cause remains to question the equal protection claim.

More important, however, there is reason to go beyond the formal similarities between donor insemination and surrogacy to their substantive differences. We can see these differences by changing our frame of reference. In highlighting their similarities we have compared donor insemination and surrogate motherhood from the point of view of the contracting couple. Seen from this perspective, the two forms of assisted reproduction may appear nearly identical. In both cases, an infertile couple turns to a third party for help in procreating a child, and the third party agrees to terminate all parental rights. Seen from the vantage point of the third party, however, things look very different, for gestating and giving birth to a child is simply not comparable to donating semen. Egg donation is more comparable, though even this procedure is considerably more burdensome and dangerous than donating semen.

When we compare the surrogate mother's role to that of the semen donor, we see a difference in kind, not just in degree. Certainly in a responsible donor insemination program a donor will be required to undergo an extensive screening process, including repeated testing for the HIV virus. But the act of providing semen itself is risk-free, nonburdensome, and simple. By contrast, the activities that the surrogate mother undertakes are neither risk-free, without burden, nor simple. Although women have rightly opposed the medicalization of pregnancy and the corresponding conceptualization of pregnancy as an illness, there can be no doubt that the physical burdens and risks of pregnancy and childbirth are so much greater than those associated with semen donation that there can be no meaningful comparison of the two. Add to these differences the emotional attachment we can expect the woman to have to her child, compared to the emotional attachment we can expect the donor to have to his semen, and we can recognize how flawed the comparison really is. Indeed, it was precisely this recognition that led the New Jersey Supreme Court to reject the Sterns' equal protection claim and to overturn the trial court's holding in this regard. As the court reasoned, even if the only difference between donor insemination and surrogate motherhood was the difference in time invested in donating sperm and carrying a child to term, there would be "more than sufficient basis to distinguish the two situations."[9] So although the Supreme Court agreed with the Superior Court that the Sterns should have custody of Baby M, it rejected the Sterns's equal protection argument and, with it, the validity of the surrogate contract.

The response of surrogacy proponents to the decision of the New Jersey Supreme Court is instructive. Although the terms of the debate are still nominally those of constitutional law, the debate itself points beyond the narrow legal questions raised by surrogacy to broader questions of morality and public policy.

Consider, for example, feminist legal scholar Lori Andrews's response to the oft-cited passage in the New Jersey Supreme Court ruling that the fact that Mary Beth Whitehead agreed to the surrogacy arrangement was irrelevant. "There are, in a civilized society," the court wrote, "some things money cannot buy." In short, there are values "more important than granting to wealth whatever it can buy, be it labor, love, or life."[10] Andrews agrees that not everything is for sale in our society, but she points out that the cases and statutes cited by the court at this point involve restrictions that apply equally to men and women. Restrictions on surrogacy, however, do not apply equally. A policy against paid surrogacy, Andrews writes, "applies disparately—men are still allowed to relinquish their parental rights in advance of conception and to receive money for their role in providing the missing male factor for procreation."[11]

We can see that Andrews is still reasoning within an equal protection framework, but notice that the real issue here is not whether the different treatment of surrogacy and donor insemination would meet the intermediate standard of review necessary to justify gender classifications.[12] Rather, it concerns what consequences follow from acknowledging that pregnancy is both an experience men cannot have and vastly different from anything men could experience in relation to donating sperm. The real issue, in other words, concerns the significance of pregnancy. In Andrews's view, to acknowledge that pregnancy is a reproductive experience unlike any other, certainly unlike donor insemination, is to open the door to systematic discrimination against pregnant women. "The other side of the gestational coin," she writes:

> . . . is that with special rights come special responsibilities. If gestation can be viewed as unique in surrogacy, then it can be viewed as unique in other areas. Pregnant women could be held to have responsibilities that other members of society do not have—such as the responsibility to have a Caesarean section against their wishes in order to protect the health of a child (since only pregnant women are in the unique position of being able to influence the health of the child).[13]

In other words, to oppose surrogacy would be to create a disparate legal category for gestation that would undermine hard-won feminist victories on other legal issues.

I believe that Andrews is properly worried that opposing surrogacy in a way that appeals to the distinctiveness of pregnancy may have some unwelcome consequences. We need only recall the recent Supreme Court case involving the fetal protection policy of Johnson Controls to appreciate Andrews's concern.[14] Acknowledging the distinctiveness of pregnancy could provide employers with a convenient justification for discriminating against women. So we must be careful in appealing to the distinctiveness of pregnancy. But the alternative to recognizing the significance and distinctiveness of pregnancy is not attractive either. It is to deny the reality of gestation in order to ensure the ideology of equality understood as equivalence.[15] Unfortunately, just such a denial underwrites the equal protection argument for surrogacy and many other arguments supporting surrogacy as well.

It is one thing to say that the law must treat men and women equally, quite another to say that it must treat them identically, even where there is substantial difference. This latter view involves an almost willful blindness to the facts of biological difference, a blindness that would be absurdly comical if it were not dangerous. When the trial court in the Baby M case compares surrogacy to donor insemination and concludes that they are essentially the same because "the donor or surrogate aids the childless couple by contributing a factor for conception and gestation that the couple lacks," it turns its gaze away from the concrete, bloody, messy reality of pregnancy and childbirth to the clean and clear-cut abstraction of "aiding the childless couple."[16] This abstraction is misleading. To describe the surrogate's role as "contributing a factor for conception and gestation" is to deny the reality of gestation and thus the reality of a woman's life.

I think that feminists and others who have opposed surrogate motherhood on the grounds that surrogacy reduces a pregnant woman to a sort of glorified container are correct. The arguments in support of surrogacy depend upon discounting the significance and distinctiveness of pregnancy.

Anti-paternalism and Pregnancy

We have seen that arguments which rely on the comparison of surrogate motherhood to DI depend upon discounting the reality of pregnancy. That is true for other arguments that support surrogacy as well. For example, the argument that surrogacy should be permitted because any state restriction would be unjustifiably paternalistic ultimately rests on a false or misleading view of pregnancy. This conclusion may not be clear at first, but a careful examination of the paternalism charge shows it to be true.

The force of the paternalism charge rests on the comparison of potential state restrictions on surrogacy to past state restrictions on women's activities that were grounded in offensive and sexist assumptions that women were incapable of making rational decisions for themselves. Ruth Macklin has put the point succinctly. The charge that surrogacy exploits women and therefore should be prohibited, she writes, "questions women's ability to know their own interests and to enter into a contractual arrangement knowingly and competently."[17] The fact that a woman may come to regret her agreement to be a surrogate or that she may agree for reasons we may not approve of is no reason to make exception to the general legal policy allowing competent individuals to provide services for a fee. Thus, to prohibit surrogacy is paternalistic and wrong.

Once again, supporters of surrogacy point to a legitimate concern. If the case against surrogate motherhood rests on the claim that women need to be protected against themselves, then prohibitions against surrogacy are indeed disturbing. If, for example, the case against surrogacy is that pregnancy produces hormonal or other biological changes in women, the force of which they can neither anticipate nor control, and that these changes set limits on the capacity of pregnant women to make or keep contracts, then the case against surrogacy is both paternalistic and thoroughly offensive. Yet the charge of paternalism misstates the case against surrogacy at this point, as we can see if we attend to the logic of the paternalism argument more closely. The charge of paternalism is premised on the assumption that surrogates are undertaking paid labor no different in kind from any other physical labor. In this view, women have a right to control what happens in and to their bodies. To interfere with this right by outlawing surrogate mother contracts is to disparage women's abilities to make rational decisions about the use of their bodies.

The argument against surrogacy, however, does not call into question women's rights to bodily autonomy, nor does it question women's decision-making capacities. Rather, the argument is that certain rights should be inalienable because to put a price on these rights and offer them for sale is essentially dehumanizing. Larry Gostin puts the point this way: "There are certain things that we can contract about—property, goods, and services. But there are other things so important to human flourishing and self-respect that they should not be specifically enforceable by contract, whether the subject is male or female."[18]

In my view, parental rights are precisely the sort of rights that should be inalienable. In particular, a woman's right to continue an intimate, caring relationship with the child she has nurtured for nine months and to whom she has given birth should not be for sale. Far from seeking to restrict a woman's right to bodily autonomy, opposition to surrogacy rather attempts to ensure that a woman's right as a parent to continue to care for her child cannot be overridden by contract. This is why I said earlier that the charge of paternalism ultimately rests on a particular (and inadequate) view of pregnancy. It should now be clear that part of the plausibility of the paternalism charge comes from the fact that it conceptualizes surrogacy as providing a service for a fee. In other words, the antipaternalists make their case by discounting both a gestating woman's relationship to the developing fetus and the way in which pregnancy involves the whole person. By focusing exclusively on the decisions a surrogate makes before she conceives, the antipaternalists draw attention from the realities of gestation and childbirth and avoid asking whether paid surrogacy is in fact dehumanizing in the way opponents say it is.

By contrast, if we attend to the actual experiences of pregnancy and childbirth, we see good reason for questioning both the picture of surrogacy painted by the antipaternalists and the practice of surrogacy itself.

For example, the surrogate contract encourages a woman to think of herself, not as a whole or complete person, but as "simply a container carrying a precious cargo that she dare not injure."[19] How else do we explain the fact that the contract Mary Beth Whitehead signed required her, among other things, to agree not "to form or attempt to form a parent-child relationship with any child or children she may conceive," nor to abort any children once conceived, nor "to smoke cigarettes, drink alcoholic beverages, use illegal drugs, take nonprescription medications or prescribed medications without written consent from her physician"? How else are we to interpret the fact that the contract required her to agree to undergo amniocentesis and to abort a defective fetus, at the request of William Stern?

But a pregnant woman is not a container, she is not an inert incubator, and to treat surrogacy as roughly comparable to letting out a room in one's home distorts the reality of pregnancy beyond recognition. To defend surrogacy, however, one has no choice but to treat pregnancy as a sort of reproductive good or service for sale. Barbara Katz Rothman has pointed out the way in which this discounts the reality of pregnancy. In the context of surrogate motherhood, she writes: "We talk openly about buying services and renting body parts—as if body parts were rented without renting the woman. But pregnancy isn't a condition of one isolated organ. Women experience pregnancy with our whole bodies."[20] We need not invoke any mystical notions about pregnancy nor infant-mother bonding to acknowledge that pregnancy is both unique and not properly described by the language of gestational services. A pregnant woman does not simply provide a womb for rent. She puts her entire body to the task of nurturing the developing fetus for nine months. Further, this physical relation often gives rise to a social relationship. For whatever mystification has surrounded notions of infant-mother bonding, many women experience a powerful identification with a child born of their bodies. Unfortunately, this is a reality that paid surrogacy obscures: Gestational motherhood is not really a service, certainly not a commodity; rather, it is a relationship.[21]

Once we acknowledge the reality of pregnancy, however, the charge of paternalism begins to appear as almost a diversionary tactic, as a way for supporters of surrogacy to change the subject when confronted with the differences between surrogacy and DI. Rather than acknowledging these differences or responding to the arguments that these differences make a difference, supporters of surrogacy take the view that the best defense is a good offense. They therefore accuse opponents of surrogacy of disparaging women by restricting their autonomy or questioning their capacities.

The case against surrogacy does not depend on treating women as insufficiently rational—because biologically impaired—during pregnancy and thus in need of state protection. Rather, in my view, the strongest argument against surrogacy rests on the conviction that certain rights recognized by the state as fundamental to human flourishing should be inalienable and that a woman's right to care for a child she has carried and nurtured for nine months is such a right. Thus, the charge of paternalism simply misses the point. The question is not primarily whether women are capable of making informed decisions about relinquishing a child prior to having conceived it, as the antipaternalists would have it. The issue is whether allowing for the sale of parental rights is so demonstrably dehumanizing and so clearly an instance of treating persons as things that we should oppose the practice.

Commodification and the Case against Commercial Surrogacy

To oppose surrogacy is not to accept paternalism; it is to reject the dehumanization of placing women and children, and the relationship between pregnant women and their children, in a cash nexus. Paid surrogacy is dehumanizing because it treats women and children as essentially fungible commodities. Consider Margaret Radin's description: "A fungible object can pass in and out of the person's possession without effect on the person as long as its market equivalent is given in exchange."[22] This definition aptly describes the view that supporters of surrogacy take of the fetus when they deny the significance of the relationship of pregnancy. So long as the surrogate is sufficiently well paid, the child can pass in and out of her possession—literally in and out of her body—without an effect on her. The woman also is treated as fungible, for one surrogate can be replaced without loss by another if she fails to conceive quickly or fails to bring to term a child quickly conceived.

Yet, as Radin points out, to treat persons as fungible objects does violence to our commonly agreed-upon view of persons as unique individuals who should be treated as ends in themselves and not simply as means to the ends of others. Because surrogacy encourages us to think of women and children as less than whole, because it encourages us to think of wombs rather than women, of characteristics that children may have rather than of the children themselves, it is fundamentally at odds with our considered views about personhood and human flourishing. The antipaternalists, of course, will respond that treating a woman as an end in herself requires respecting her autonomy and thus respecting her right to contract to be a surrogate. The problem with the antipaternalist response at this point is that it offers an impoverished account of human autonomy, one that essentially equates freedom and alienability in markets. Indeed, we can see that in the antipaternalist view all rights are treated as roughly analogous to property rights that can be bought and sold in markets, and freedom is seen as the individual's ability to maximize wealth by trading in markets. In this view, the problem with paid surrogacy is that any restriction on a woman's ability to enter a contract is a fundamental violation of her autonomy and her freedom to maximize her economic interests.

Once again, however, Radin has pointed out how fundamentally at odds such a conception of freedom is with our considered views about personhood. Indeed, Radin has offered a devastating critique of the attempt to cast all human interaction in market terms. To adopt market rhetoric to describe human interactions or to adopt a market methodology to assess these interactions is to view human life from an alien perspective, one that most of us would reject upon close examination. Radin attempts to show that this is the case by examining an example of the attempt to understand noneconomic activity in market terms. The example she chooses is Richard Posner's analysis of laws against rape. The example is extreme, but useful nonetheless. Posner says that rape should be conceptualized as the theft of a property right: "The prohibition against rape is to the marriage and sex 'market' as the prohibition against theft is to explicit markets in goods and services."[23] In other words, we need laws against rape to protect a woman's right to offer her body (i.e., her self) for trade, whether in marriage (or in noncontractual sexual relations) or in prostitution, just as we need laws against theft to ensure the stability of markets in general.

As Radin points out, to talk about rape in these terms is to treat bodily integrity as "an owned object with a price." The problem is that we simply do not think of ourselves in these terms. It is not a woman's *body* that has been raped; it is *she*. The violation of bodily integrity, in other words, is deeply personal in a way that simply cannot be accounted for in market terms. As Radin puts it, "We feel discomfort or even insult, and we fear degradation or even loss of the value involved, when bodily integrity is conceived of as a fungible object."[24]

Not only does market rhetoric misdescribe rape from the point of view of the victim, it is also inadequate to describe rape from the point of view of the rapist. As usual, to speak in market terms will be to use the language of cost-benefit analysis and thus to speak of rape as benefiting the rapist, as indeed Posner does. Yet, under what plausible account of human flourishing could rape possibly be understood to benefit the rapist? The answer is clearly none. We are led to conclude that to try to account for all human actions in market terms is to adopt an inadequate account both of personhood and of human flourishing.

In drawing on Radin's critique of Posner, I do not mean to suggest that the antipaternalist is *necessarily* committed to accepting an economic analysis of rape or a similarly crude analysis of surrogate motherhood. Rather, the point is to highlight the fact that in opting for a view of freedom as negative liberty and defining liberty as the ability to relinquish rights for a fee, the antipaternalist will be hard-pressed to offer an analysis of surrogacy that does not echo Posner's treatment of rape. Thus, we should not be surprised to discover that the antipaternalist view depends in part on discounting the significance of pregnancy to the surrogate by seeking to separate the woman from the womb, much as Posner's analysis turns on detaching a woman from her body and treating it as impersonal property. The problem in both cases is that to undertake the necessary separation requires us to deny a recognizable and real human experience: on the one hand, the rape victim's sense of personal violation, on the other hand, the surrogate's experience of relating to the fetus.

By contrast, if we acknowledge the way in which pregnancy engages the whole person and we refuse to define freedom narrowly as the liberty to sell anything for a price, then restrictions on surrogacy will cease to appear paternalistic. On the contrary, eliminating surrogacy may be seen as enhancing freedom in that it fosters respect for a woman's bodily integrity that is understood not as owned property but as a deeply personal matter central to human flourishing. Here we see clearly that equal protection arguments rely on discounting the significance and distinctiveness of pregnancy, just as antipaternalism arguments do. Indeed, we can now see that the antipaternalist shares with the equal protection supporter of surrogacy the view that surrogacy is essentially similar to donor insemination. Both treat gestating and giving birth to a child as involving no greater personal and emotional involvement than providing semen in a lab, and both therefore believe that paid surrogacy is acceptable. Indeed, both disparage pregnancy and are frequently united in the view that surrogacy is comparable to DI. This disparagement of pregnancy explains why supporters of surrogacy so frequently compare surrogacy to DI. For both, surrogacy is a service, not a relationship. Both ignore the fact that gestation differs profoundly from semen donation and that the surrogate's relationship to a child is utterly unlike the semen donor's relationship to a child.

Once we acknowledge the relationship that pregnancy involves, however, we see that we cannot move too quickly from an assessment of DI to an assessment of surrogate motherhood. To be sure, surrogacy shares a number of things in common with DI, so some of the considerations that we raised in the last chapter will be relevant here as well. For example, both surrogacy and DI separate genetic and social parenthood by introducing third-party gametes into the process of procreation. Thus, the problems raised for DI by secrecy and asymmetry will be raised for surrogate motherhood as well. We can expect, for example, that to keep the truth from a child born through surrogate motherhood will have the same corrosive effects on the family unit as does secrecy in DI. We can expect, too, that the fact that the child's father is both the genetic and social father while his spouse is only the social mother will introduce tensions into the marriage and into the mother's relationship with the child about which we must be concerned. Nevertheless, if we consider just the similarities between surrogate motherhood and donor insemination, we might reach the same conclusion about surrogacy as we did about DI: Although it is problematic and not for everybody, it may be morally acceptable, so long as it is not undertaken in secret.

The Differences Make a Difference

I have suggested, however, that we must not look just to the similarities between surrogacy and donor insemination—we must attend to their differences as well. We have seen that perhaps the most fundamental difference is that surrogacy involves a relationship with a child in a way that donor insemination does not. At best, we might say that the semen donor has a relation to the resulting child, but a relation of genetic connection is not a relationship of care. Providing gametes to assist in the conception of a child is not equivalent to caring for and nurturing a developing fetus for nine months. Nor is the relation of genetic connection likely to ground an emotional attachment to the fetus in the way gestational relation often does. Nor does donor insemination involve a commitment of the whole person in the way that surrogacy clearly does. Although the donor admittedly may—and ideally would—consider his sperm to be a personal gift, the gift does not require a sustained physical and emotional commitment. Thus, donating sperm does not promote the sort of detachment from embodied existence that surrogacy, understood as a gestational service, requires.

When we consider these differences in light of our previous discussion of responsible parenthood, we see that we cannot treat surrogacy as morally equivalent to donor insemination. We have seen that when we compare the distinct activities of begetting a child and rearing one, we should assign priority to the latter, not the former. If we ought to assign greater moral significance to the "social" activities of parenting than to genetic connection, it follows both that a surrogate mother's parental role is more important than that of a surrogate father's, and that when a conflict arises between a surrogate mother and a contracting father over parental rights and responsibilities, the surrogate's claim at least initially should be given greater weight. In other words, if the activities of caring for and rearing a child are constitutive of parenthood in a way that simply begetting a child is not, the gestational mother must be considered a parent to the child she carries. Although gestating a child is not rearing a child in any full social sense, it is closer to the activities constitutive of parenthood than is begetting a child or contracting to have a child conceived.

This is not to say that the contracting father is incapable of caring for the child as well as the gestational mother. It is, rather, to highlight the fact that the child's father is not yet a social parent and thus has not demonstrated the same level of commitment as the gestational mother. I realize that to assign the gestational mother priority on this basis is to turn a temporal difference, i.e., the fact that the surrogate is the first individual to care for the child, into a moral prerogative.[25] That is true but justified. It is not mere temporal difference that is here assigned moral significance. Rather, I wish to assign priority to the rearing component of parenthood, and unless we ignore reality, we must acknowledge and respond to the fact that only women rear children in their bodies.

If I am right that parenthood is constituted primarily in the activities of nurturing a child, i.e., in relationship, then a surrogate mother is unquestionably a parent of the child, even in the case where the child is not the genetic offspring of the surrogate. If the relationship makes the parent, the decision to become a surrogate is the decision to become a parent. To repeat: At the very least the surrogate will have a nurturing relationship with the fetus she carries; often she will have much more, including a developing emotional relationship with it. This last point is likely to be overlooked if we hold either of two views. If we believe that the fetus is not a person, we are likely to dismiss the possibility that a pregnant woman can have any meaningful emotional relationship with the fetus she carries. Alternatively, if we believe that it is possible to choose not to form a relationship with the developing fetus, then we may hold the view that (social) parenthood is avoidable simply through an act of the will.

I do not believe that either view is plausible. Even if we wish to deny—as I do—that the fetus is a person from conception, even if we insist on distinguishing between a "fetus" and a "child" for much of the pregnancy, at some point it will not be plausible to make this distinction and to insist that the fetus is not a person. At some point, the surrogate mother is carrying a child with whom something more than a physical relationship is possible. Nor is it plausible to suggest that the surrogate may simply choose not to enter the relationship. As David H. Smith has pointed out, when humans interact with animate beings over time, they tend to become personally involved, whether we are talking about "4-H kids and livestock, or a researcher and a mouse tested over several months."[26] Can we reasonably suppose that a woman could knowingly have the most intimate interaction with a fetus for nine months and not form a relationship with the fetus?

When we thus ask of surrogate motherhood the same question we ask of donor insemination—Will a child conceived through this form of assisted reproduction be properly cared for by its parents?—we get a different answer. When we ask this question in the case of surrogate motherhood, we will not be inquiring simply about the contracting couple but about the surrogate mother as well. Is she capable of meeting the demands of parenting, and can we reasonably expect the fetus/child to flourish in her care?

Supporters of surrogacy try to avoid questions of this sort when they talk about the surrogate as a provider of a service rather than as a parent. To admit that the surrogate is a parent is to invite an assessment of her parenting; it is to acknowledge that she may parent well or badly and that gestating a fetus/child well requires commitment.

By contrast, once we acknowledge that to become a surrogate is to become a parent, we also begin to see more clearly what is wrong with surrogacy and why it is not morally on a par with donor insemination. Surrogacy requires us either to deny the parental relationship of the surrogate to the child or to treat this relation instrumentally, as transferable for a price. That is why I think George Annas points to a central difficulty with surrogacy when he notes that surrogacy "can create one parent-child relationship only by destroying another parent-child relationship."[27] Here we glimpse a hidden but disturbing truth about surrogacy: In undertaking surrogacy, the surrogate mother creates a parent-child relationship with the intention of severing it.

The surrogate contract, of course, obscures this fact because it seeks to frame the mother's relationship to the child she carries as supervenient upon the father's relation to the child, as if the surrogate's relationship to the child were somehow a function of the father's consent. Thus, for example, the contract that Mary Beth Whitehead signed stipulated that she would not form a parent-child bond with any child she conceived. This attempt to create a legal fiction, however, does not change the reality of pregnancy. Every mother is engaged in social interaction with her fetus, whether the pregnancy is wanted or not.[28] The fetus will make demands on her, and she will respond. She may be joyful or resentful, she may angrily try to deny its existence, or she may give the fetus a nickname and talk to it regularly, but she is unlikely to be distant from the fetus in the way that the language of surrogate contracts implies.

Given that the surrogate mother will have a parent-child relationship with the fetus she carries, we must ask whether such a relationship can be responsibly undertaken when the surrogate is expected to perceive her responsibility to the fetus solely as an artifact of her contractual relation to the biological father and his spouse.[29] Notice that this question is not applicable in the case of donor insemination, because the donor is not responsible for the care of the fetus in the way that the surrogate unavoidably is, and thus in providing sperm the donor is not, even implicitly, making a commitment to care. By contrast, because the surrogate will necessarily care for the fetus, it is reasonable to ask about the grounding for that care. How committed can we expect the surrogate to be to the care of her child? In most cases, the answer is likely to be that the surrogate is only marginally and provisionally committed. On her own, she does not wish to conceive a child; she does not plan to raise the child; she even agrees not to bond with the child. Under these conditions can we expect a surrogate properly to care for the child?

When we add to these considerations the fact that the surrogate is paid to enter into a parental relationship with the fetus she carries—though as we saw, the contract obscures this fact—and to end that relationship for a price, we see how instrumentally surrogacy treats the parent-child relationship. The problem with commercial surrogacy is thus not simply that it requires a woman to treat her bodily integrity as owned property available for sale to a buyer, but also that it places human relationships, indeed, one of the most intimate human relationships, in the marketplace. And the problem with commercializing relationships is that truly committed, caring relationships are not something we can simply buy and sell. The prospect of buying or selling a friend, for example, is both repugnant and ultimately impossible. It is repugnant because to suggest that one could rent a friend as one rents, say, a car debases the value we place on friendship; it is impossible because someone who agreed to be a "friend" for a price would not in fact be a friend.

That is not to say that those who are paid to care for others cannot genuinely love those whom they help, but to the extent that paid caregivers do genuinely love, they will have placed more importance on the relationships they have with their charges than on the goods they receive in payment for their services. Here Nel Noddings's distinction between types of caring is illuminating. According to Noddings, we should distinguish between two types of caring. "Caring-for," in Noddings's view, is a full-bodied reciprocal relationship with the "cared-for" that includes an emotional attachment to, and identification with, the "cared-for." It typically involves a "displacement of interest" and a movement of the caregiver away from the self toward the reality of the other. By contrast, "caring-about" is a thin and wan relationship. It does not involve emotional attachment; there is no displacement of self-interest; indeed, one needn't even know the person for whom one is caring.[30]

If an ideal of genuine caring is caring-for, then we will expect parents to care-for their children because, at the very least, responsible parenthood involves genuine caring. Unfortunately, commercial surrogacy, at least, is at odds with genuine caring because the relationship of the surrogate to the child is made secondary to the contract and is valued only instrumentally as something for which the surrogate will be paid. Indeed, if Noddings is correct about what genuine caring involves, we could even say that the surrogate is paid *not* to care for the child. As we have seen, the surrogate agrees not to form an emotional attachment to, or a relationship with, the child.

The case of noncommercial surrogacy is less clear. I can certainly imagine a case in which a woman whose own children fill her life with joy and who treasured the experience of being pregnant offers to be a surrogate for a childless friend. Such an offer might indeed come from a desire to ease the pain of her friend by providing a gift of great value. To be sure, such a case is significantly different from the typical commercial transaction of surrogacy. We cannot say of the surrogate in this case that she values her relationship with the fetus/child only instrumentally, that she values the child only for what she receives in payment for it. Nor can we say that surrogacy in this case places human relationships in the marketplace. It is precisely because the surrogate values her relationship to her friend so highly and because she appreciates the importance of the parent-child relationship itself that she is willing to be a surrogate. Thus, she values pregnancy and the child that results independently of financial rewards or incentives.

Nevertheless, even unpaid surrogacy requires a sort of emotional schizophrenia that is at the very least troubling. She is supposed to care for the child she carries, yet maintain the requisite emotional distance to be able to relinquish the child at birth. So even here difficult questions about instrumentalization arise. The surrogate's relationship to the fetus is still contingent upon the father's desire to have a child through the use of her body, and she must not allow herself to think or feel entirely otherwise.

The question we ought to put to any form of assisted reproduction, including surrogacy and donor insemination, is whether there is something about conceiving a child in this way that conflicts with the very purpose for which responsible parents conceive children. When we ask this question of surrogacy, we get a decidedly different answer from that given in relation to donor insemination. Because surrogacy requires a mother to attempt to maintain an emotional distance from the fetus she carries, because it demands that she regard the child as belonging only to the biological father and his spouse, and because it treats her relationship to the child as parasitic upon her agreement with the biological father, surrogacy is fundamentally in conflict with the commitment to care that is at the heart of responsible parenthood.

One objection to my argument at this point will certainly be that the only reason I reach different conclusions about donor insemination and surrogacy is because I pose the question to different parties in these two contexts. In the case of donor insemination, I ask whether the procedure conflicts with the commitment and ability of the contracting couple to care, but not the donor, whereas in surrogacy I ask the question of both the contracting couple and the surrogate.

Admittedly I draw this distinction, and noting it highlights what I have suggested throughout this chapter, namely, that one's view of surrogacy depends in large measure on whether one thinks it is like or unlike donor insemination. I have argued that surrogacy is fundamentally unlike donor insemination because the surrogate has a relationship with the child, is a parent to the child, in a way that a sperm donor does not and is not. I have also suggested that to deny the difference is to deny the reality of pregnancy and thereby to deeply discount its significance and uniqueness. Yet if we acknowledge the reality of pregnancy, if we attend to the relationship between the surrogate and the child, then we see why we must ask whether the circumstances of conception conflict with the surrogate's commitment to care for the child, even though we do not ask this question of the sperm donor. The fact of the matter is simply that the donor occupies a different moral space than the surrogate in relation to the child conceived through these two forms of assisted reproduction. She has a relationship to the child that he does not. Consequently, we must judge the two cases differently.

Focusing on this relationship helps us to see, for example, why paying a surrogate is so much more troubling than paying the semen donor. We have seen the trouble with commercial surrogacy. By placing human relationships in a cash nexus, paid surrogacy treats women and children as fungible commodities and is thus essentially dehumanizing. By contrast, because providing sperm does not involve establishing a relationship with a child, paying a "donor" is not yet to commercialize human relationships. That is not to say that paying for sperm ought to be encouraged. On the contrary, in my view, a system of voluntary sperm donation would be greatly preferable to the current system (in the United States) of paid donation. Still, there is a difference between paying for sperm and paying for pregnancy and, once again, the difference has to do with the creation of a caring relationship.

Although this fundamental difference is clear, we should not lose sight of the fact that similarities also exist between surrogate motherhood and donor insemination and that these similarities underwrite the attempt by supporters of surrogacy to use the acceptance of donor insemination as a sort of fulcrum by which to raise commercial surrogacy to respectability. We should keep this fact in view because it helps us to appreciate that the concerns raised in the first three chapters (that reproductive technology would first commodify reproduction and then commercialize it) were not baseless. That is not to say that I now think better of slippery slope arguments. On the contrary, I hope my argument has shown that we can draw serious moral distinctions among various forms of reproductive technology and that to accept one form is not to accept every form. Nevertheless, having seen how a comparison to donor insemination is used in an attempt to legitimate surrogate motherhood, we can also appreciate why some opponents of reproductive technology have wanted to draw the line very conservatively between acceptable and unacceptable reproductive interventions. For these writers, the risk of accepting any form of assisted reproduction is real, and it grows with each successive level of intervention until the point where third-party gametes are involved, at which point all forms of assisted reproduction are beyond the pale and each is disastrous.

Armed with this conviction that most forms of assisted reproduction are unnecessary because there is, in adoption, a perfectly acceptable and morally unproblematical alternative to assisted reproduction, critics of reproductive technology typically have opposed reproductive interventions altogether or have drawn the line of acceptable forms of assisted reproduction at the use of third-party gametes. I have tried to show throughout this volume that both these critical perspectives are mistaken. In doing so, I have called into question the conviction that there is a threshold level of intervention beyond which we must not go. By contrast, I have tried to show that we must consider each form of assisted reproduction, each new application of reproductive technology, as it comes. There is, in other words, no unstoppable snowball effect, and there is nothing to be gained by drawing boundaries in relation to abstractions such as "use-of-third-party-gametes" or the like.

On the contrary, much is to be learned from asking how a particular form of assisted reproduction affects or will affect the relationships of the parents to the children. I ask this question repeatedly throughout this volume, albeit in different forms. By treating reproduction merely functionally, does DI contribute to parents relating to their children improperly as investments rather than as gifts? Will the loss of intimacy in conceiving a child through assisted reproduction result in a loss of intimacy between the parents and a child so conceived? Can prospective parents responsibly undertake parenthood when there is some risk of creating a child who will suffer as a result of the way in which he was conceived? Can we properly care for our children when the means by which they are created involves conceptualizing them as objects? Can we expect the relationship of a father to a child to be fully loving when she is conceived through the union of the gametes of his spouse and a third party? Can we expect a mother to properly care for her child when she conceives not out of love but for money? These are the sorts of questions that I believe must be answered if we are to reach an adequate view of assisted reproduction, and thus I have tried to answer some of these questions at length. Yet there is another question that I have not addressed as I have tried to articulate the boundary of acceptable forms of assisted reproduction. Though frequently left unstated by critics of reproductive technology, the question haunts many discussions of assisted reproduction. Why bother? Why pursue reproductive technology when there is adoption?

The forcefulness of the question emerges when the question itself is fully stated. Given the tremendous cost and effort associated with reproductive technology, given the potential dangers, the possible harm to children, the risk of commodifying reproduction, how can we justify creating children through assisted reproduction when children already in existence do not have parents to care for them? In short, given that assisted reproduction is so morally ambiguous, how can we justify using it when we could adopt instead? Although this question cannot easily be dismissed, it gains much of its power from the conviction that adoption is morally unproblematic. It is this conviction that I take up in the next chapter.

Part III

Adoption and Reproductive Technology

6

The Myth and Reality of Current
Adoption Practice

When I have outlined this book for friends and colleagues, the first question has almost always been, Why adoption? What place does adoption have in a book on assisted reproduction? Certainly that is a reasonable question. After all, most of this volume has concerned issues raised by a technology that is relatively new, exotic, and designed to create life. Adoption, by contrast, is not new; it involves no exotic technology and responds to a life already in existence. So, indeed, why adoption?

The answer to this question harks back to a point I made at the start of the volume. Assessments of reproductive technology are not made in a vacuum. Forms of reproductive intervention are assessed, at least in part, in light of the available alternatives. Adoption is an alternative. To be sure, adoption does not offer the prospect of genetic or gestational parenthood as other forms of assisted reproduction do, but it does offer what I have argued is the central experience of parenthood, namely, the ongoing, day-to-day task of caring for and nurturing a child. So adoption is an alternative to reproductive technology that must be considered.

Rhetorical Uses of Adoption

The fact that adoption is an alternative to *in vitro* fertilization, donor insemination, and surrogate motherhood is important. Critics of these forms of assisted reproduction often rely on a comparison to adoption to bolster their case against the offending reproductive intervention. Yet, whether explicit or merely implicit, the comparisons to adoption almost always assume that adoption is morally unproblematic. Therein lies the force of the comparison: given that surrogate motherhood, say, is so potentially damaging to all the parties involved, why pursue surrogate motherhood when you can adopt and thereby redress harm rather than cause it?

The problem with such comparisons is that adoption is left unexamined—hence, this chapter. When we take a closer look at adoption, we see problems with the institution that I believe force us to reassess the comparisons between adoption and other forms of assisted reproduction and to rethink adoption as an alternative for infertile couples. This chapter, then, asks whether adoption is as morally unproblematic as most critics of other forms of assisted reproduction appear to assume. The answer, I suggest, is that it is not. In saying this I do not mean to suggest that those who have pursued parenthood through adoption have done something wrong. Nevertheless, if we are to make any meaningful assessment of adoption as an alternative to reproductive technology as a means of pursuing parenthood, we have no choice but to examine adoption honestly and directly. When we undertake such an examination, we discover that current adoption practice in this country is characterized by the same trends toward commodification and commercialization that we have worried about throughout this volume. We will see that there are other problems as well.

To see how the comparison to adoption functions in an assessment of reproductive technology, and why such comparisons are problematic, let us turn to an examination of donor insemination in which the comparison to adoption is explicitly used to disparage DI. Consider an article written by the philosopher David N. James, which takes up various objections to DI that have been raised.[1] James considers and rejects these objections, including those based on natural law and concerns about overpopulation. Although James believes that most of the standard objections to donor insemination are flawed, he argues that there is one overwhelming argument, which compares donor insemination to adoption. Indeed, he calls the argument the "Adoption Objection."

James begins by identifying the need to which we are attempting to respond in treating infertility. There are, he says, various desires at work when persons seek infertility treatment. Some persons desire genetic offspring; some persons desire the experience of gestating a child; some desire the experience of caring for and nurturing a child; and some desire all of these together. Nevertheless, says James, the only desire we ought to try to meet is one based on a legitimate interest or need: the desire to nurture.

According to James, if this need is what we seek to redress, adoption is morally preferable to DI. We can see this, says James, by comparing the ways in which adoption and DI meet this need. When successful, donor insemination, like adoption, provides a child for a couple who have a legitimate interest in nurturing a child. DI, however, does not produce the other social benefits that adoption does. Adoption relieves society of the cost of caring for unwanted children, donor insemination does not; adoption enriches the lives of unwanted children, donor insemination does not; adoption helps the problem of overpopulation, donor insemination does not. James frames the argument in syllogistic fashion.

1. Couples who seek artificial insemination have a morally justified fundamental interest in becoming parents.

2. But adoption of existing orphaned or unwanted children allows couples to satisfy this fundamental interest in becoming parents.

3. Adoption of orphaned and unwanted children enriches their lives, relieves society of the expense of their care, and promotes the goal of limiting population, and thus has several social benefits.

4. Practices which produce social benefits and allow satisfaction of the fundamental interests of individuals are preferable to practices that satisfy individual's interest without producing such social benefits.

5. AID does not produce the social benefits which adoption does.

6. Therefore, adoption is preferable to AID.[2]

James's argument here amounts to a paradigm of the type of comparison that stands behind much criticism of *in vitro* fertilization, donor insemination, and the like. Although James is much more explicit than most critics in comparing reproductive technology to adoption, the basic reasoning is the same. Given that adoption helps unwanted children, saves the taxpayers money, and serves the goal of population control, how could we possibly justify the expense, the diversion of resources, or the possible harm of undertaking exotic reproductive interventions?

What should we make of this argument? Whatever force the argument has, it gains from the unexamined assumption that adoption is morally unproblematic. Perhaps it is a given that adoption helps unwanted children and that donor insemination does not. But, even so, it does not follow that adoption is without its problems. Once we acknowledge this fact, it should be clear that nothing at all follows from James's argument and certainly not that adoption is preferable to donor insemination. Even in a strictly utilitarian calculus, we must examine the costs as well as the benefits before we could reach such a conclusion, and this James does not do.

Indeed, like most others who make the comparison between adoption and donor insemination, James says virtually nothing about the actual practice of contemporary adoption or, for that matter, about donor insemination. The only concession he makes to the reality of adoption practice comes in response to an anticipated objection to his argument. He says that some may respond to his argument by noting that fewer children are available for adoption today than previously and that, consequently, infertile couples who now wish to adopt face a longer wait and a more stringent screening process. For James, this reality appears scarcely relevant. As a response to his adoption objection, he says the concern about long waits is "wholly inadequate." "While it is wrong to violate the fundamental interests of individuals to promote desirable social goals," he writes, "there is nothing wrong with asking people to defer for some period of time the satisfaction of their fundamental interest. . . . The proper reply to couples who object to the long wait required to adopt is that they should learn the virtue of patience."[3]

James's acknowledgment that the number of children available for adoption has declined reveals that he is not unaware of the realities of contemporary adoption; nevertheless, the passage quoted above betrays an acute myopia to the meaning of this reality. For the declining number of healthy white infants available in this country for adoption through authorized agencies has meant, not just longer waits for prospective parents, but, among other things, a fundamental shift in adoption practice toward private and international adoptions. We will see shortly that this shift is important and must be taken into account in assessing adoption as an alternative to other forms of assisted reproduction, and this is worrisome if nothing else. Thus to say so glibly that fewer infants and longer lines simply demand greater patience is to reveal not merely an insensitivity to the suffering of the infertile but a sort of moral stupor to the significant facts about contemporary adoption.

The Reality of Current Adoption Practice

If we are fully to assess the comparison of adoption to other forms of assisted reproduction, we must attend in much greater detail to the realities of current adoption practice in this country and to their moral significance. I have already indicated that I plan to draw attention to some of the more troubling aspects of that practice, but it is also important to point out why adoption typically receives such unqualified support. The reason is simply that there exists a laudable tradition of support for adoption in this country as an appropriate means of providing for the welfare of unwanted, abused, or orphaned children. Unlike adoption in other places and in other times, in this country adoption has, at least since the passage of the first adoption legislation in the United States in 1851, always been properly oriented to securing the welfare of children who need parents. Indeed, even when adoption practice has been seen primarily as a service for childless couples—as it has at times in this century—it has not lost its focus on the welfare of children in need.[4] So there is good reason to support adoption as a practice that serves the needs of innocent children. Indeed, at first glance, adoption appears well suited to respond to the needs of all involved in the so-called adoption triangle without harm to anyone. Birth parents who are unable to care for their child can relinquish that child for adoption with confidence that he or she will be properly cared for; infertile couples receive the child they cannot have otherwise; and, most significantly, an unwanted child receives a good home. So, again, there appears to be good reason for supporting adoption.

At the same time, however, we must also ask where adoption practice stands today. We can begin to answer that question by noting that it is customary to distinguish types of adoption according to the sorts of intermediaries involved in placing the child and according to the country of origin of the child adopted. The typical picture of adoption, of course, is that of a child born in this country placed through a nonprofit, public, and licensed agency with a childless couple whom the agency has deemed suitable parents for the child. In return for the agency's services, the adoptive couple pays a modest fee and, after a probationary placement period, a judge formalizes the adoption by decree.

This, however, is not the only, or even the most common, form of adoption today, at least not for infertile couples. In addition to public adoption agencies, there are private agencies and private individuals that serve as intermediaries to adoption placements; there are for-profit agencies as well as nonprofit agencies; and there are children born abroad who are adopted by individuals and couples in this country, again through various types of intermediaries. So the practice of adoption in the United States today presents a complicated picture. There are public domestic adoptions, private agency domestic adoptions, private or "independent" domestic adoptions, private agency foreign adoptions, and private individual foreign adoptions. And the trend is toward independent, domestic adoptions and international adoptions. In 1975, for example, independent adoptions accounted for 8.5 percent of children placed for adoption in this country; in 1986 that number was 15.4 percent. In 1975, 5,633 children from abroad were placed for adoption in this country; in 1987 there were 10,097 such placements. Indeed, in just the period 1985–1987 foreign adoptions increased 8.7 percent in the United States.[5]

What is the significance of such trends? To answer that question we must consider the differences between various types of adoption. Consider, for example, the differences between public agency adoptions and independent adoptions. We have already sketched the common perception of public agency adoptions, and the perception fairly matches the reality. Public adoption agencies are typically subsidized by state welfare programs and are thus able to place children for adoption at a cost far below the actual expenses involved for prenatal, hospital, counseling, and legal fees usually associated with adoption. According to the National Committee for Adoption (NCFA), the usual range of costs for adopting for a public agency is $0–$3,000, with the median being $1,000.[6] Public agencies typically have professionally trained social workers who act as liaison for all the parties involved with the adoption. They also typically provide counseling services to birth mothers and prospective parents, and they screen prospective parents for psychological problems that would interfere with successful adoptions. Public agencies usually conduct home studies and discuss the subject of telling children about adoption with prospective adoptive parents.

In contrast, consider the independent adoption. Strictly speaking, an independent adoption is any in which a licensed agency does not participate in placing the child.[7] So any adoption in which prospective parents and birth mothers are brought together without the help of an agency would count as an independent adoption. Physicians, nurses, or family friends sometimes bring together birth mothers and prospective parents, but typically independent adoptions are arranged by attorneys for a fee. Independent adoption is considerably more expensive than public agency adoption. Rather than a range of $0–$3,000, independent adoption is $2,000–$20,000, with a median of $12,000.[8] Unlike public agency adoptions, independent adoptions rarely involve trained social workers as intermediaries and the attorneys do not screen the prospective adoptive parents. In many independent adoptions there is no home study before the child is placed, and according to one study of independent adoptions, home studies for independent adoptions are cursory compared to those for agency adoptions.[9] According to a NCFA survey, fewer than half of those lawyers arranging independent adoptions discuss the subject of how best to tell a child he or she is adopted.[10]

Consider, too, the way in which birth mothers are recruited for independent adoptions. One common practice is for the brokering attorney to place advertisements in the classified section of newspapers on behalf of his clients. Below are two fairly typical ads of this sort.

> BABY WANTED: Please help us find a baby to adopt. Childless couple love children dearly and can provide a good loving home. Well educated, own our own home, good jobs, and lots of love to give. PLEASE, PLEASE HELP US. WE HAVE TRIED EVERYTHING! CONTACT OUR ATTORNEY.

> ADOPTION. Young, white, well-educated, financially secure, happily married couple. We cannot conceive a child and desperately want to adopt a newborn. Our promise to your baby—EVERY ADVANTAGE THAT LIFE HAS TO OFFER but most of all LOTS AND LOTS OF LOVE. We will provide financial help with all medical bills, legal fees, food, housing, maternity clothes, and counseling if desired.
> PLEASE THINK ADOPTION.
> CONFIDENTIAL. CALL COLLECT.[11]

When we consider that about 50 percent of all domestic adoptions of healthy infants are independently arranged, and that public agency placements account for only about 5 percent of such adoptions, we can begin to see the mistake of treating public agency adoptions as the model for all adoptions. Indeed, even using public agency adoptions as the paradigm for all agency adoptions is misleading, for while 45 percent of domestic adoptions of healthy infants are handled through private agencies, there are substantial differences between private and public agencies. For example, in 32 states it is possible for a private for-profit organization to be licensed as an adoption agency, and surely the practices of a for-profit agency will be different from those of a nonprofit agency.[12]

Just as we cannot make generalizations about domestic adoptions on the basis of practices of public adoption agencies, neither can we generalize about foreign adoptions on the basis of reputable, nonprofit private agency international adoptions. There are private for-profit agencies arranging international adoptions, and private individuals both here and abroad acting as intermediaries for international adoptions.

Once we recognize the mistake of holding up public agency adoptions as the model of all, foreign or domestic, we see, too, why we cannot speak about adoption as an alternative to reproductive technology while ignoring the realities that do not measure up to that ideal. And the distressing truth of the matter is that the reality of many current adoption practices is far from ideal. Consider just the practices associated with independent adoption. We see here many of the same problems we have worried about elsewhere in this volume. We have worried, for example, about the commercialization of reproduction that seems to follow from the introduction of expensive, high-tech methods of conceiving a child, and of the commodification of children that may be encouraged by the high price tags on the children conceived through reproductive medicine. We have worried about a system that appears driven by the desires of prospective parents and that does not appear to safeguard the interests of the children desired by those parents. Should we not be equally concerned about the obvious commercialization of soliciting birth mothers through financial incentives and of paying brokers tens of thousands of dollars to arrange private adoptions? Should we not be equally concerned that the high cost of independent and foreign adoptions exert the same pressures towards commodification of children as do the high costs of reproductive technology? Should we not be equally concerned that, like reproductive medicine, current adoption practice is being driven by the demands of the desperately infertile without sufficient attention being paid to the welfare of children?

The obvious answer to all of these questions is that we certainly should be concerned about the direction in which adoption is moving. My point, however, is not to disparage adoption so much as it is to show why the comparison of reproductive technology to adoption is flawed. Indeed, I think we can now see one reason why variations of what David James calls the "adoption objection" to reproductive technology appear persuasive. Opponents of reproductive technology rarely discuss the reality of adoption when they make the comparison. When we look at the reality of adoption, the so-called adoption objection seems hardly to be an objection at all.

The Comforting Myth of "Unwanted Children"

The comparison of reproductive technology to adoption is not flawed merely by what James and others choose not to discuss; the way that adoption is discussed is also problematic. Consider once again James's argument for the superiority of adoption over donor insemination. Recall that his basic point is that adoption produces social benefits ameliorating the laws of adoptive children. Hence the third step in his argument: "Adoption of orphaned and unwanted children enriches their lives, relieves society of the expense of their care, and promotes the goal of limiting population, and thus has several social benefits." Notice the use of the language of "orphaned and unwanted children." In one sense, such language is as misleading as failing to discuss the changing situation of contemporary adoption practice. Such language conjures images of abused and battered children and of bad parents. Adoption is thus made to seem not merely socially useful but salvific. Yet while there are surely abused and battered children who are rescued through adoption, we should not ignore the social reality that creates "unwanted children" in an effort to add a gloss of moral excellence to adoption. Indeed, even to talk about "unwanted children" may be misleading in situations where a woman is relinquishing a child not because she is *unwilling* to care for her child, but because she is *unable* to do so. The fact that in both situations the child will be labeled "unwanted" should give us pause about assuming that adoption unambiguously serves the needs of all the parties in the adoption triangle.

It seems to me that any honest assessment of adoption must take into account the reasons for which women relinquish children for adoption. To speak about "unwanted children" is to fail to take seriously what is perhaps the most compelling reason women relinquish children, namely, poverty. In the blinkered view taken by James, "unwanted children" are obviously abandoned by "selfish mothers" who care more about their career than their kids. The reality, of course, is much more complex.

Consider, for example, the situation of international adoption. Perhaps it is here that the notion of "unwanted children" is most transparently misleading. There is little pretense that foreign women relinquish children for reasons other than economic and political oppression. Indeed, it is part of the mythology of international adoption that such adoptions are commendable precisely because a child is being rescued from what is almost surely a life of poverty and destitution. A review of the major countries of origins of children adopted in the United States also supports this view. In the fiscal year 1987, for example, the following countries relinquished the greatest number of children for adoption in the United States: Korea, India, Colombia, Philippines, Guatemala, Chile, Mexico, Brazil, El Salvador, and Honduras. Significantly, when we compare the number of children adopted from such generally impoverished and politically unstable areas with those from more prosperous, stable areas, the contrast is striking. For example, although 7,614 children born in Asia were adopted in the United States in the fiscal year 1987, and 2,017 were brought from Central and South America during that year, only 122 came from Europe.[13]

Nor should we assume that mothers relinquish children for economic and political reasons only in international adoptions. Although the evidence is clearer with international adoptions, there is reason to believe that fear of poverty is a significant motivating factor for American women who surrender children for adoption. For example, in a study of the experiences of 334 parents who gave up children for adoption, Eva Deykin, Lee Campbell, and Patricia Patti found that "external factors, including family opposition [to keeping the child], pressure from physicians or social workers, and financial constraints, were cited by 69 percent of the sample as the primary reason for surrender."[14] Similarly, in his study of mothers who relinquished children for adoption, Edward K. Rynearson found that "all of the subjects perceived relinquishment as an externally enforced decision that overwhelmed their internal wish for continued attachment to the baby."[15] Or consider a study by George Burnell and Mary Ann Norfleet of eighty women who placed their children for adoption: nearly two-thirds of the women had not completed high school, "nearly half reported incomes under $6,000, and only 6 percent made over $15,000 per year."[16]

Although such data are not conclusive, Deykin, Campbell, and Patti are surely correct when they observe that renewed pro-life efforts to restrict access to abortion combined with cuts in social services and financial aid to unmarried single women exert significant pressure on poor and uneducated women to "choose" the adoption option.[17] Indeed, when we consider that the number of children living in poverty is now estimated to be 14 million, and that three-quarters of the newly homeless are thought to be families with children, it would be surprising if women were not relinquishing children for adoption in order to avoid the appalling fate of the homeless in this country.[18] In short, it may be profoundly misleading to describe children placed for adoption as "unwanted."

Nor is it simply the description "unwanted" that may be inaccurate, for the fate of homeless parents also suggests that the category of "abused" children may mislead. For example, in his book on homeless families in America, Jonathan Kozol describes the way in which children of homeless parents may be classified as "abused" for the simple reason that they are enmeshed in an inadequate social service system. He writes:

> A welfare mother who has no home and has yet to locate shelter runs another risk of being separated from her child. A lawyer in Los Angeles describes a scenario repeated daily in America: A homeless family applies for AFDC. The social worker comes to the decision that the children are endangered by their lack of shelter. The children are taken away and placed in foster care. The parents are no longer eligible for AFDC now because they don't have children. So the family as a family receives nothing. The children have been institutionalized. The family, as such, exists no longer.[19]

Moreover, as Kozol points out, there are incentives for parents to relinquish children built into the system.

New York will spend a great deal less to support an AFDC child in the home of her real mother than to subsidize that child in a foster home. A twelve-year-old child living at home in New York City is allocated a maximum of $262 a month for all food, clothes, and rent expenses (1986). If this child were taken from her mother for "abuse or neglect," the child would then be allocated $631 monthly.[20]

Once we acknowledge that women often relinquish children out of economic necessity, we see the flaw in arguing that adoption is preferable to donor insemination because it rescues unwanted children and donor insemination does not. The flaw is that many children surrendered for adoption are not in fact unwanted by their biological parents, but are relinquished anyway because there is no alternative. To acknowledge this fact is also to acknowledge that adoption does not unproblematically serve the interest of all parties in the adoption triangle as is commonly supposed. On the contrary, we can now see that adoption may often benefit the adoptive parents at the expense of the biological parents, particularly birth mothers.

Adoptive Parents Versus Birth Parents

Although little attention has been paid in the past to the experiences of birth mothers after they relinquish a child, there is increasing evidence that surrendering a child for adoption is deeply traumatic and that the trauma is long lived. In addition to the studies by Deykin, Campbell, and Patti; Rynearson; and Burnell and Norfleet just cited, there are at least two other frequently cited studies of the experience of relinquishing a child for adoption that reached the same conclusions: surrendering mothers mourn the loss of children given up for adoption, sometimes their whole lives. Many feel they had no choice, but nevertheless regret the decision. Many have experienced negative effects on subsequent parenthood, including overprotectiveness, compulsive anxiety about their children's health, and difficulty accepting their children's increasing independence. Indeed, the summary offered by Robin Winkler and Margaret van Keppel of their study of the long-term adjustment of relinquishing mothers nicely summarizes most of the literature on this topic. According to Winkler and van Keppel, "the effects of relinquishment on the mother are negative and long lasting," and "relinquishing mothers, compared to a carefully matched comparison group of women, had significantly more problems of psychological adjustment."[21]

Given the view of pregnancy I defended in chapter 5, the relinquishing mothers' sense of loss should come as no surprise. If the experience of pregnancy is not discounted, if, as I argued, pregnancy involves the development of the relationship between the mother and the fetus that is the precursor to the full-blown social relationship that defines parenthood, then we should not be surprised to learn that to sever that relationship, whatever the reason, is deeply traumatic. Indeed, we can now see that the discussions of adoption are frequently flawed by the same two mistakes that I have argued flaw discussions of donor insemination and surrogate motherhood: the significance of pregnancy is too easily dismissed and parenthood is treated as a sort of zero-sum game.

I argued in chapter 4, for example, that when thinking about the moral wisdom of intentionally separating genetic and social parenthood there is a tendency to pose a stark either/or. Either the genetic mother and father are the real parents, or the social mother and father are; they cannot all be the parents of the child. We see the same tendency in discussions of adoption. Since adoption advocates see a preoccupation with genetic connection as an obstacle to a more widespread acceptance of adoption, they are inclined to the opposite view, namely, that genetic parenthood has no significance. They therefore insist that the adoptive parents are the "real" parents, thereby effectively reducing the genetic parents to nonentities.

In fact, we can now see that treating parenthood here as a zero-sum game goes hand in hand with discounting the importance of the pregnant woman's relationship with the developing child. If the point of the system is to facilitate the placement of a child, and if the adoptive mother must be seen as the child's real mother in order to ensure that such placements go smoothly, we will need to avert our gaze from the relationship between the relinquishing mother and her child. If we focus on their relationship for long, it may appear too real to deny. So we focus instead on the adoptive parents rather than on the woman who has given nine months of her life to nurture a child and who may not be all that keen on surrendering it.

I see no more reason to suppose that we must pit genetic and social parents against one another here than in cases of donor insemination. In other words, we may define parenthood primarily in social terms and nevertheless value the genetic contribution of the biological parents and acknowledge their role as parents. Moreover, as we saw in chapter 5, if we define parenthood primarily socially, we will not be inclined to discount the significance of the relationship between a birth mother and her child. Unfortunately, because discussions of adoption typically presuppose a stark choice between genetic and social parents, and because the relationship between birth mothers and their children is frequently ignored, the moral ambiguity of adoption is itself obscured. Adoption is thought to be an unqualified good.

Rhetoric versus Reality

We can now see that the picture of adoption as an unqualified good is not entirely accurate. We must face the fact that there are human costs to adoption and that every adoption involves loss. As Barbara Katz Rothman puts it, "When we think of adoption, that is what comes to mind: the waiting arms, the welcoming parents. But for every pair of welcoming arms, there is a pair of empty arms. For every baby taken in, there is a baby given up."[22]

Once we focus on the grief and sense of loss of birth mothers, my earlier suggestion that relinquishing a child for adoption may be a coerced decision may not seem so implausible. At the very least I think we can now see that current adoption practices raise troubling issues of race and class. Once again Barbara Katz Rothman nicely summarizes the problem:

> If we step outside the psychological dynamics of adoption, if we look for a moment at the class relations in adoption, some ugly facts emerge. "Poor countries export children to rich ones, black parents to white, poor parents to better off." And if we take a thoughtful look at the mechanisms established for facilitating adoption, we can also accurately say that "adoption agencies are a system for redistributing children from the poor to the middle classes." Thirty-two-year-old attorneys living in wealthy suburbs do not give up their children to nineteen-year-old factory workers living in small towns. Whether we look at the birth mothers who go through adoption agencies and compare them with the adoptive couples who go home with their babies, or look at the open marketing of babies as practiced via newspaper ads and brokers, we see that adoption is as much a class issue as it is anything else.[23]

In short, when we take a close look at adoption, we see that the rhetoric does not match the reality. The conventional piety is that adoption facilitates the interests of all parties to the practice—birth parents, adoptive parents, and children; that it safeguards society from the corrupting practice of trafficking in children; and, most importantly, that it is oriented toward, and serves well, the interests of the children placed for adoption. We have seen, however, that adoption does not always serve the interest of all the parties involved; that, at the very least, the system often takes advantage of a particularly vulnerable group of women in order to satisfy the desires of a far less vulnerable group; and that in the trend toward independent and international adoption, the institution itself begins to appear decidedly commercial. So there is reason to be less than reverential about adoption. Indeed, it seems to me that we must even question the most sacred dogma of adoption advocates: Is the institution of public agency adoption itself in fact oriented toward, and does it serve, the best interest of the child?

The answer to that question, I believe, is that agency adoption is designed and does serve the interest of adoptive children, on the whole. Yet even the system's commitment to the best interest standard is more equivocal than might initially be supposed. Consider, for example, the response of the Child Welfare League of America (CWLA) to transracial adoption over the past thirty or forty years. The CWLA is the most influential and prestigious group of adoption professionals in this country, and, as its name suggests, the group identifies the welfare of adoptive children as its primary goal. Nevertheless, the CWLA's position on transracial adoption has changed several times since the 1950s in ways that appear inconsistent with the commitment to pursuing the best interest of adoptive children.

Writing in the *Notre Dame Law Review*, Margaret Howard has chronicled the changes in the positions of the CWLA.[24] In 1958, the CWLA's *Standards for Adoption Service* set out a somewhat equivocal position on transracial adoption. Although transracial adoption was discouraged, it was not categorically opposed. According to the CWLA, "physical resemblances should not be a determining factor in the selection of a home, *with the possible exception of such racial characteristics as color.*" By 1968, the CWLA was actively encouraging transracial adoption. "It should not be assumed by the agency or staff members that difficulties will necessarily arise if adoptive parents and children are of different racial origin. . . . In most communities there are families who have the capacity to adopt a child whose racial background is different from their own. Such couples should be encouraged to consider such a child." In addition, the clause from the 1958 standard identifying racial characteristics as a possible exception was dropped. By 1972, the CWLA had changed its position again. Once more, the CWLA had become ambivalent about transracial adoption. "While we specifically affirm transracial adoptions as one means of achieving needed permanence for some children, we recognize that other things being equal in today's social climate, it is preferable to place a child in a family of his own racial background."[25]

What explains the CWLA's changing position on transracial adoption? One explanation is surely that the CWLA has appropriately calibrated its position on transracial adoption to the dramatic changes in race relations in this country during the past thirty years. Using a best interest standard, it may well have been the case that discouraging transracial adoption was wise in the volatile years of the late fifties and early sixties. Moreover, by 1968, race relations may have appeared sufficiently evolved that it seemed in the best interest of prospective adoptive children to endorse transracial adoption. But why the change from 1968 to 1972? And why does the CWLA still say that "children in need of adoption have a right to be placed in a family that reflects their ethnicity or race"?[26]

The answer has to do, in part,[27] with the fact that in 1972 the National Association of Black Social Workers (NABSW) condemned the adoption of black children by white parents as a "form of genocide." As Howard points out, "available evidence suggests that wholesale adoption by whites of black or mulatto children has never occurred,"[28] and thus the charge of genocide was nonsense. Nevertheless, the NABSW had legitimate concerns. They were worried that a black child raised by white parents would not be prepared for the racism he or she would inevitably confront in our society. They were concerned that black children raised by white parents would lose their cultural identities and indeed might have no sense of themselves. So certainly the NABSW, and the CWLA following them, had the best interest standard guiding their decisions to a degree.

Nevertheless, as the charge of genocide would seem to indicate, other political and ideological commitments were at work here. Indeed, a closer look at the 1972 statement by the NABSW shows that concern for the welfare of individual children was certainly not the primary goal. "We have taken the position," the NABSW writes,

> that black children should be placed only with black families whether in foster care or for adoption. Black children belong, physically, psychologically and culturally in black families in order that they receive the total sense of themselves and develop a sound projection of their future. Human beings are products of their environment and develop their sense of values, attitudes and self concept within their family structures. Black children in white homes are cut off from the healthy development of themselves as black people. Our position is based on:
> 1.   the necessity of self determination from birth to death, of all Black people.
> 2.   the need of our young ones to begin at birth to identify with all Black people in a Black community.
> 3.   the philosophy that we need our own to build a strong nation.[29]

Two items in particular from this statement suggest that the NABSW is not acting on the basis of a best interest standard. When the association talks about the healthy development of adoptive children as "black people," and when their position is justified in relation to the goal of building a "strong [black] nation," it seems clear that the position is not articulated with the interest of the individual children as the most central goal.

That condemning transracial adoptions could not be in the interest of black children can be seen by considering what the alternatives are to transracial adoption. Since there are nowhere near the number of black families waiting to adopt as there are black children needing adoption, the alternatives are foster care or placement in an institution. Yet there is a general consensus that the uncertainty of foster care placements and the absence of a continuous caring relationship with a specific adult caregiver with institutional placement make foster care and institutionalization poor substitutes for adoption. So to condemn transracial adoption is to condemn children to forms of care that are known to be inadequate. Indeed, in the year before the NABSW condemnation of transracial adoption there were 2,574 black-white adoptions; in 1972 there were 1,569. Perhaps the development of those 1,000 children as "black people" was safeguarded by avoiding transracial adoption, but their development as people was unlikely to have been.

As Howard points out, "The weight of clinical data and psychological opinion supports the conclusion that foster care and institutionalization are seriously detrimental to the emotional development of affected children."[30] Moreover, Howard also argues that the studies of the emotional development of transracially adopted children suggest that transracial adoptions are successful, even in terms of the issues of racial identity raised by the NABSW. Indeed, one study she cites found that "both white and non-white children raised in mixed-race families were less likely to have pro-white attitudes or to associate 'white' with positive and desirable characteristics than were both white and non-white children generally."[31]

Nor is Howard alone in questioning the opposition to transracial adoption. Elizabeth Bartholet, for example, has argued persuasively that "today most public and private adoption agencies are governed by powerful race matching policies" and that such placement policies adversely affect black children.[32] As Bartholet demonstrates, whether we look at state and federally funded subsidies to facilitate inrace adoption of minority children, agency policies that require holding black children in foster care for a time if no same-race family is available, or differential screening criteria favoring black families seeking to adopt, there is unmistakable evidence of system-wide opposition to transracial adoption. And the result of such opposition is that potential adoptive homes are denied to black children, even when the upshot is that such children will never find permanent homes.

In defending transracial adoption, I do not mean to suggest that transracial adoption is problem-free. We live in an intensely race-conscious, and frequently racist, society. Some transracially adopted children will suffer as a result. Some children may well be plagued by identity issues. Some white parents will be unprepared to address the special needs of a black child adopted by white parents, and the child will suffer as a result. On the whole, however, it seems clear that applying a best interest standard would lead to active endorsement of transracial adoption, particularly when the alternatives are foster care or institutionalization. So why has the CWLA not endorsed transracial adoption? The only possible answer it seems to me is that the CWLA is not following a best interest standard.

Although even the institution of public agency adoption does not always serve the best interest of children needing adoption, this does not mean that the system for placing children for adoption is badly flawed or even that the system needs to be substantially changed. My point is rather that the system is not perfect and that there are pressures on the system that work against the best interest of the child. Any complete assessment of adoption would acknowledge as much.

Unfortunately, when critics of reproductive technology compare forms of assisted reproduction to adoption, they do not typically bother with an examination of adoption. They do not discuss the reality, but only the mythology of adoption. They do not acknowledge the ever present danger of coercion with adoption; they do not acknowledge the troubling issues of class and race at work; they do not acknowledge the increasing blurring of the distinction between buying a baby and acquiring one through independent adoption. If critics of reproductive technology were to acknowledge these facts about contemporary adoption, they probably would not be so sanguine about comparing reproductive technology to adoption. Indeed, once we take a close look at adoption, it becomes clear that pursuing parenthood through adoption requires the same moral vigilance that I have urged for pursuing parenthood through the use of reproductive technology. As with other forms of pursuing parenthood, adoption cannot be unequivocally endorsed or condemned. As with other forms of pursuing parenthood, adoption must not be undertaken lightly or without attending to the difficult moral issues it raises.

Epilogue

Critics of assisted reproduction often point to the fact that the treatment of infertility does not respond to any medical need. Infertility, they say, is not a disease; it is neither life threatening nor particularly debilitating. Indeed, even when infertility impairs proper biological functioning, it rarely imperils health. So the question arises, how can we justify spending a billion dollars a year on infertility treatment when basic health care needs are not being met? In one sense, this is a reasonable question to which there is no good answer. At least there is no good answer if you believe—as I do—that infertility treatment is important because it provides individuals with access to a basic human good, the good of raising children. Yet I suspect that even for those who confront infertility and who want nothing more than to have their own children, the choice between providing for the very real medical needs of children who already exist and meeting the needs of the infertile would not be a difficult one. If we are forced to choose, for example, between IVF and inoculations for children, we should obviously choose inoculations. This suggests that posing such a choice is not particularly helpful in thinking about assisted reproduction. This is even more apparent when the choice is said to be between the needs of a particular group of patients and the desires of the infertile. Need is contrasted with desire to make infertility treatment appear morally on a par with cosmetic surgery. In this view, IVF becomes a sort of rhinoplasty for the ego.

In my view, this is a profoundly misleading view of infertility and, like so many other criticisms of assisted reproduction, this line of attack distracts us from the central issues we need to address. To be sure, infertility treatment frequently responds more to a desire than to a medical need. But we need to ask about the nature of this desire. Although the desire is complex, its most basic object is typically that of nurturing a child, and the realization of this desire ought to be constrained by the goal toward which the desire ultimately moves, namely, the well-being of the child in one's care. Seen in this light, the desire to have children should not be trivialized by comparison with cosmetic surgery. On the contrary, the desire to care for a child ought to be deeply respected as a basic human good.

At the same time, we must also acknowledge that such a desire is not one that should be met at all costs or one that can be met in only one way. I have tried to show, for example, that parenthood may be pursued in ways

135

that are fundamentally incompatible with the desire to nurture a child, at least where this includes putting the child's well-being before one's own. So the desire to have children is neither trivial nor ultimate, and the pursuit of parenthood through assisted reproduction to which this desire gives rise should not be unconditionally embraced or utterly rejected. Perhaps, ultimately, such a conclusion is, as my colleague gently but derisively suggested, properly characterized as "ample interventions, always with tears." If so, my hope is that the sorts of moral concerns to which I have drawn attention in this volume, and which could easily give rise to heartache and tears, may sometimes shape the actions of the infertile and their caregivers before as well as after the pursuit of parenthood.

NOTES

Introduction

1. U.S. Congress, Office of Technology Assessment, *Infertility: Medical and Social Choices, OTA-BA-358* (Washington: Government Printing Office, May 1988).

2. Leon Kass, *Toward a More Natural Science* (New York: Free Press, 1985), p. 101.

3. See, for example, Sidney C. Callahan, "The Role of Emotion in Ethical Decisionmaking," *Hastings Center Report* 18/3 (June/July 1988): 9–14, as well as her book, *In Good Conscience: Reason and Emotion in Moral Decision Making* (San Francisco: Harper, 1991).

4. Robyn Rowland, "Women as Living Laboratories: The New Reproductive Technologies," in *The Trapped Woman*, ed. Josefina Figueira-McDonough and Rosemary Sarri (Newbury Park: Sage, 1987), pp. 81–111.

5. Gena Corea, *The Mother Machine* (New York: Harper and Row, 1985).

6. Nancy Ann Davis, "Reproductive Technologies and Our Attitudes towards Children," *Logos* 9 (1988): 51–77.

7. Kass, *Toward a More Natural Science*, p. 45.

8. I am, in effect, suggesting that more choice is not always better than less. This is not a popular view in our culture, but it can be persuasively defended. For such a defense, see Gerald Dworkin, "Is More Choice Better than Less?" in *Social and Political Philosophy* (Minneapolis: University of Minnesota Press, 1982): 47–61. Dworkin quotes Kierkegaard to good effect in this essay: "In possibility everything is possible. Hence in possibility one can go astray in all possible ways" (47).

9. It is important to note here that although IVF was a potential option for overcoming my infertility, it was not primarily a treatment involving me. Some feminist critics have been opposed to IVF to treat male infertility for this reason: a woman who is perfectly fertile is subjected to the trauma of IVF for a problem that is not her own. Although this is a legitimate concern, to be categorically opposed to the use of IVF to treat male infertility is to be blind to the way a couple may see infertility as a common problem, even though only one of them is infertile. The fact that both individuals may be treated, although only one is infertile, also means that the worries about guilt and blame that I just noted may be lessened in some cases.

10. The only exception to this concerned one experimental technique for treating male-factor infertility that my urologist opposed.

11. See John Rawls, *A Theory of Justice* (Cambridge: Harvard University Press, 1971), pp. 48–51, and "The Independence of Moral Theory," *Proceedings and Addresses of the American Philosophical Association* 47 (1974/75): 5–22. Also see Norman Daniels, "Wide Reflective Equilibrium and Theory Acceptance in Ethics," *Journal of Philosophy* 76 (1979): 256–82. In his later work Rawls draws a distinction between narrow and wide reflective equilibrium. What I describe here is wide.

12. Rawls, "The Independence of Moral Theory," *Proceedings and Addresses of the American Philosophical Association* XLVII (1974/1975), p. 8.

13. Morton White, *What Is and What Ought To Be Done: An Essay on Ethics and Epistemology* (New York: Oxford University Press, 1981).

14. White has sometimes been interpreted as suggesting that we cannot revise our feelings about particular moral conclusions, that feelings are incorrigible. Regardless of where White stands on this point, I reject it. In my view, a recalcitrant moral response to a particular moral conclusion can lead us to reconsider moral and

descriptive beliefs that went into reaching the conclusion, but it can also lead us to reconsider our moral feelings. Change is possible in either direction, in my view. This is why I said earlier that personal experience is not incorrigible.

15. *What Is and What Ought To Be Done*, p. 30.

16. Ibid.

17. It is important to say here, however, that we may also need to revise our feelings in such a situation. This is a possibility that White does not always hold clearly in view.

18. Bernard Williams, *Ethics and the Limits of Philosophy* (Cambridge: Harvard University Press, 1985), p. 94.

19. Williams restricts spontaneous convictions to "moderately reflective but not yet theorized" beliefs. My use of the term is thus wider than Williams's, for I would also include emotions.

20. Michael Tooley, "Abortion and Infanticide," *Philosophy and Public Affairs* 2/1 (Fall, 1972): 39. Tooley takes a somewhat more charitable view of such intuitions in his later book by the same name. See *Abortion and Infanticide* (Oxford: Clarendon Press, 1983), pp. 24–30.

21. This is not to say that these responses are incorrigible. I agree with Jeff Stout that "the myth of the given is as naïve and misleading in morals as it is in science." See Stout, *Ethics after Babel* (Boston: Beacon Press, 1988), p. 157.

22. H. Tristram Engelhardt, Jr., *The Foundations of Bioethics* (New York: Oxford University Press, 1986), p. 9.

23. Congregation for the Doctrine of the Faith (Washington, D.C.: U.S. Catholic Conference), Publication no. 156-3 (hereafter cited as *Instruction*).

24. Paul Ramsey, "Abortion: A Review Article," *The Thomist* 37/1 (January 1973): 174-226, at 205.

1. Dualism and Disembodiment?

1. Here I mean interventions that involve the manipulation of gametes.

2. U.S. Congress, Office of Technology Assessment, *Artificial Insemination Practice in the United States: Summary of a 1987 Survey* (Washington: Government Printing Office, 1988).

3. On this point, see John A. Robertson, "Embryos, Families, and Procreative Liberty: The Legal Structure of the New Reproduction," *Southern California Law Review* 59 (1986): 942–1035.

4. The cases from which Justice White is quoting here are *Meyer v. Nebraska*, *Skinner v. Oklahoma*, and *May v. Anderson*.

5. William E. May has offered a similar interpretation of the reasoning of the *Instruction*, although we disagree dramatically about the adequacy of the reasoning. See his "Catholic Moral Teaching on *In Vitro* Fertilization," in *Reproductive Technologies, Marriage and the Church*, ed. Donald G. McCarthy, (Braintree, MA: Pope John Center, 1988), pp. 107–21.

6. *Instruction*, p. 26.

7. The Vatican here quotes from Pope Pius XII, "Discourse to Those Taking Part in the Second Naples World Congress on Fertility and Human Sterility," May 19, 1956, *AAS* 48 (1956): 470.

8. *Instruction*, p. 32.

9. Ibid., p. 27.

10. The emphasis on the symbolic dimension of embodiment found in this part of the document is at odds with the heavily biological interpretation of natural law theory found elsewhere in the *Instruction*. On this contrast see James Nelson, *Embodiment: An Approach to Sexuality and Christian Theology* (Minneapolis: Augsburg, 1978), p. 28.

11.   Lisa Sowle Cahill, "Women, Marriage, Parenthood: What Are Their 'Natures'?" *Logos* 9 (1988): 19.

12.   For a response to this claim about the objectification of reproductive medicine, see Robertson, "Embryos, Families, and Procreative Liberty," p. 1024.

13.   I thus agree with Richard McCormick's claim that the Instruction "is more concerned with contraception than with reproductive technologies. If the Church's analysis of contraception were different than it is, the document would be substantially different." From "Document Is Unpersuasive," *Health Progress* 68 (July-August 1987): 53.

14.   *Instruction,* p. 29.

15.   McCormick has pointed out that failure to attain "proper perfection" is not equivalent to being morally wrong, although the Vatican here so construes it. "The Vatican Document on Bioethics: Two Responses," *America* 156 (March 28, 1987): 248.

16.   On this point, see Richard McCormick, "Document Is Unpersuasive," 55, and Edward V. Vacek, "Notes on Moral Theology: Vatican Instruction on Reproductive Technology," *Theological Studies* 49 (1988): 114–15.

17.   "The Theological Report of the Papal Commission on Birth Control," June 26, 1966, in *Love and Sexuality,* comp. Odile M. Liebard (Wilmington, NC: Consortium Books, 1978).

18.   "Theological Report," p. 302.

19.   Ibid., pp. 302–3; emphasis added.

20.   Ibid., p. 304.

21.   Ibid., p. 305.

22.   It is important to note that there is not one but several feminist responses to reproductive technology. Indeed, feminist responses range from enthusiastic support (Shulamith Firestone's *The Dialectic of Sex* (New York: Morrow, 1970)) to moderate and cautious support (some of the essays in the collection *Reproductive Technologies: Gender, Motherhood and Medicine,* ed. Michelle Stanworth (Minneapolis: University of Minnesota Press, 1987)) to radical opposition (the essays in *Made To Order,* ed. Patricia Spallone and Deborah Lynn Steinberg (Oxford: Pergamon Press, 1987)).

23.   Gena Corea, "The Reproductive Brothel," in *Man-Made Women,* Gena Corea et al. (Bloomington: Indiana University Press, 1987), p. 39.

24.   Barbara Katz Rothman, "The Products of Conception: The Social Context of Reproductive Choices," *Journal of Medical Ethics* 11 (1985): 191.

25.   "First Human Gene-Therapy Test Begun" *Science News* 138/12 (September 1990): 180.

26.   John A. Robertson, "Genetic Alteration of Embryos: The Ethical Issues," in *Genetics and the Law III,* ed. Aubrey Milunsky and George Annas (New York: Plenum Press, 1985), p. 118.

27.   Germ line gene therapy, however, may be considerably more difficult than somatic gene therapy. On this point, see Fred D. Ledley, "Somatic Gene Therapy for Human Disease: Background and Prospects," *Journal of Pediatrics* 110/1–2 (January/February 1987): 1–8, 167–74.

28.   Shelley Minden, "Patriarchal Designs: The Genetic Engineering of Human Embryos," in *Made to Order,* p. 105.

29.   Jalna Hanmer, "Transforming Consciousness: Women and the New Reproductive Technologies," in *Man-Made Women,* p. 105.

30.   Janice Raymond, "Fetalists and Feminists: They Are Not the Same," in *Made to Order,* pp. 61–62.

31.   Anne Donchin, for example, has persuasively argued that utopian visions of a future in which women are liberated from the burdens of childbearing through reproductive technology have never gained widespread support within feminism because such visions are always unacceptably dualistic. Writing about the views of

perhaps the best-known advocate of such technological liberation, Shulamith Firestone, Donchin says that her views rest "on conceptual foundations that have much in common with the presuppositions and policymakers who would pursue goals antagonistic to her own, who would support technological intervention for the sake of the monopoly of power it would make possible. Both sorts of interests view technology as a victory over nature. . . . Both see human biology as a limit to be overcome." See "The Future of Mothering: Reproductive Technology and Feminist Theory," *Hypatia* 1/2 (Fall 1986): 130.

32.   Msgr. Carlo Caffara has argued that it is opposition to this instrumental relationship between one's intentions and one's body that underlies the Roman Catholic church's rejection of artificial insemination. See "The Moral Problem of Artificial Insemination," *Linacre Quarterly* 55/1 (February 1988): 38.

33.   On this point, see Cahill, "Women, Marriage, Parenthood," p. 20.

34.   Joseph A. Selling has also pointed out that understanding the full unity of the human person requires us to recognize not only the bodily and spiritual dimensions of our existence but our historicity and relatedness to the material world and others. "The Instruction on Respect for Life: II. Dealing with the Issues," *Louvain Studies* 12 (1987): 323–61.

35.   Actually, there are at least three different techniques being investigated. See Jon W. Gordon et al., "Fertilization of Human Oocytes by Sperm from Infertile Males after Zona Pellucida Drilling," *Fertility and Sterility* 50/1 (1988): 68–73. Also see Soon-Chye Ng, Ariff Bongso, Sheau-Ine Chang, et al., "Transfer of Human Sperm into the Perivitelline Space of Human Oocytes after Zona-Drilling or Zona-Puncture," *Fertility and Sterility*, 52/1 (1989): 73–78.

36.   In fact, it was my doctor, who had moral reservations about this technique, who first pointed this out to me.

37.   Moreover, the drive to develop reproductive technology is clearly fueled by financial incentives. Nothing perhaps illustrates this more clearly than the development of an embryo flushing technique by a team of physicians at Harbor-UCLA Medical Center. In April 1983, this team successfully flushed an embryo from one woman and transferred it to a second woman, who carried the fetus to term. The project was funded by Fertility and Genetics Research, a for-profit company begun by two physicians who envisioned the establishment of a chain of embryo transfer clinics where infertile women could purchase embryos to gestate themselves. Indeed, to ensure themselves the maximum profits, the Harbor-UCLA team sought to patent the equipment and their technique (see Corea, *The Mother Machine*, esp. chap. 6).

38.   Davis, "Reproductive Technologies," pp. 51–77.

39.   Ibid., p. 57.

40.   Ibid., p. 58. Joseph Selling has suggested that the Vatican itself is guilty of this privatization of procreation. See Selling, "Instruction on Respect for Life," pp. 335–36.

41.   Davis, "Reproductive Technologies," p. 56.

42.   Jonathan Hewitt, "Preconceptional Sex Selection," *British Journal of Hospital Medicine* 37 (February 1987): 151–55.

2. Commodification and Coercion

1.   *Instruction*, p. 21.

2.   Patricia Spallone, *Beyond Conception* (London: Macmillan, 1989), 59; Anita Direcks, "Has the Lesson Been Learned? The DES Story and IVF," in *Made to Order*, pp. 161–65.

3. Paul Ramsey, *Fabricated Man* (New Haven: Yale University Press, 1970). p. 113. He is writing here specifically about ectogenesis, but the point applies to IVF as well.

4. For a review of what we do know about the risks of IVF, see J. D. Schulman, J. D. Paulson, A. Dorfman, and M. I. Evans, "Genetic Aspects of IVF," in *Foundations of In Vitro Fertilization,* ed. Christopher M. Fredericks, John D. Paulson, and Alan H. DeCherney (Washington, D.C.: Hemisphere, 1987).

5. Direcks, "Has the Lesson Been Learned?" p. 164.

6. Spallone, *Beyond Conception,* p. 89; also see Kass, *Toward a More Natural Science,* p. 52.

7. Spallone, *Beyond Conception,* p. 93.

8. Ibid., p. 96.

9. As quoted in B. E. Carey's "Informed Consent by Participants: Who Participates? Who Consents?" in *Test-Tube Babies,* ed. William A. W. Walters and Peter Singer (Melbourne: Oxford University Press, 1982), p. 66.

10. Kass, *Toward a More Natural Science,* p. 114.

11. On this point, see Rowland, "Women as Living Laboratories"; Lucile F. Newman, "Framing the Ethical Issues in New Reproductive Technologies," *Health Care for Women International* 8 (1987): 287–92.

12. On this point, see Alison Jaggar, *Feminist Politics and Human Nature* (Totowa, NJ: Rowman and Allanheld, 1983), p. 210.

13. See Barbara Katz Rothman, *Recreating Motherhood: Ideology and Technology in a Patriarchal Society* (New York: W. W. Norton, 1989), p. 62.

14. See Brigitte Jordan and Susan L. Irwin, "The Ultimate Failure: Court-ordered Caesarean Section," in *New Approaches to Human Reproduction: Social and Ethical Dimensions,* ed. Linda M. Whiteford and Marilyn L. Poland (Boulder, CO: Westview Press, 1989), pp. 13–24.

15. Spallone, *Beyond Conception,* p. 67.

16. As quoted in Rothman, *Recreating Motherhood,* p. 62.

17. *Women's Studies International Forum* 8/6 (1985): 547–48.

18. "Women as Living Laboratories," p. 85.

19. Kass, *Toward a More Natural Science,* p. 25.

20. "Newborn Screening for Sickle Cell Disease and Other Hemoglobinopathies," *National Institutes of Health Consensus Development Conference Statement* 6/9 (April 6–8, 1987). I owe this example to Val Flechtner.

21. It is important to point out, however, that Ramsey's argument was not just that IVF may harm fetuses, but that it wrongs them. Thus, he was concerned with the issue of respect as much as with that of damage.

22. Derek Parfit, *Reasons and Persons* (New York: Oxford University Press, 1986), pp. 351–55.

23. Robertson, "In Vitro Conception and Harm to the Unborn," *Hastings Center Report* 8 (October 1978): 13–14.

24. See, for example, E. Haavi Morreim, "Conception and the Concept of Harm," *Journal of Medicine and Philosophy* 8 (1983): 137–57.

25. Kass, *Toward a More Natural Science,* p. 55.

3. The Expanding Market

1. U.S. Congress, Office of Technology Assessment, *Infertility: Medical and Social Choices, OTA-BA-358* (Washington: Government Printing Office, 1988), p. 305.

2. American Fertility Society, "Ethical Considerations of the New Reproductive Technologies," *Fertility and Sterility* Supplement 46/3 (1986): 26s–28s.

3. Ibid., p. vii.
4. Ibid., pp. 27s–28s.
5. Ibid., p. 31s.
6. Ibid., p. vii.
7. Ibid., p. 29s.
8. *Junior L. Davis v. Mary Sue Davis,* 1989 Tenn. App. Lexis 641, 14. For an account of property that might allow for preimplantation embryos to be personal property but not fungible, see Margaret Jane Radin, "Property and Personhood," *Stanford Law Review* 34 (May 1982): 957–1015. It is also worth pointing out that in June 1992 the Supreme Court of Tennessee overruled the trial court and held that Junior Davis could prevent his former wife from using their frozen embryos. In so ruling, the Supreme Court of Tennessee followed AFS guidelines by referring to the frozen cells as preembryos, but it refused to define them, strictly speaking, as either persons—as the trial court had—or as property—as the appeals court had. See "Court Gives Ex-Husband Rights on Use of Embryos," *New York Times,* 2 June 1992, National Edition, p. A1, col. 2.
9. John A. Robertson, "The Right to Procreate and In Utero Fetal Therapy," *Journal of Legal Medicine* 3/3 (1982): 333–66.
10. Robertson, "Procreative Liberty and the Control of Conception, Pregnancy, and Childbirth," *Virginia Law Review* 69/3 (1983): 416.
11. Robertson, "Embryos, Families, and Procreative Liberty: The Legal Structure of the New Reproduction," *Southern California Law Review* 59 (1986): 958.
12. As quoted in "Embryos, Families, and Procreative Liberty," p. 959.
13. Robertson, "Procreative Liberty and the Control of Conception," pp. 408–9.
14. Ibid., p. 410.
15. Ibid., p. 406.
16. Robertson, "Embryos, Families, and Procreative Liberty," p. 961, n. 69.
17. *Infertility: Medical and Social Choices,* pp. 251–52.
18. Robertson, "Procreative Liberty and the Control of Conception," pp. 433–34.
19. Ibid., p. 403.
20. Robertson, "Embryos, Families, and Procreative Liberty," p. 990.
21. Ibid., p. 988.
22. Kass, *Toward a More Natural Science,* p. 113.
23. Robertson, "Embryos, Families, and Procreative Liberty," p. 1024.
24. Robertson, "Gestational Burdens and Fetal Status: Justifying *Roe v. Wade,*" *American Journal of Law and Medicine* 13/2–3 (1988): 200.
25. Robertson, "Embryos, Families, and Procreative Liberty," p. 966.
26. Robertson, "Technology and Motherhood: Legal and Ethical Issues in Human Egg Donation," *Case Western Reserve Law Review* 39/1 (1988–89): 1–38.
27. Robertson, "Technology and Motherhood," p. 31.
28. Robertson, "Rights, Symbolism, and Public Policy in Fetal Tissue Transplants," *Hastings Center Report* 18/6 (December 1988): 7.
29. Robertson, "Embryos, Families and Procreative Liberty," p. 975.
30. The contrast Blackmun draws is between "an unlimited right to do with one's body as one pleases" and a right to privacy. Whether he means to suggest that the right to bodily autonomy does not bear a "close relationship" to the right of privacy or whether only an unlimited right to bodily autonomy does not do so is unclear.
31. Robertson, "Gestational Burdens and Fetal Status: Justifying *Roe v. Wade,*" *American Journal of Law and Medicine* 13/2–3 (1988): 193.
32. Robertson, "Rights, Symbolism, and Public Policy," p. 8.
33. Ibid., p. 8; emphasis added.
34. Even here, though, I think a case can be made that aborting the fetus is not to *use* the fetus.

35. Robertson, "Embryos, Families, and Procreative Liberty," pp. 971–75.
36. We have seen, for example, that Robertson testified in the Davis case that the preimplantation embryo should be treated as fungible property.
37. Robertson, "Procreative Liberty and the Control of Conception," p. 410.
38. Robertson, "Embryos, Families, and Procreative Liberty," pp. 964–65.
39. Kass, *Toward a More Natural Science*, p. 110.
40. Rothman, *Recreating Motherhood*, pp. 29–47.
41. Strictly speaking, if paternity is the central relationship, genetic connection to the father is all that matters. But as Rothman points out, historically in the West, the basic idea concerned the importance of the seed, and this idea has been retained by extending the concept to women. So the basic idea behind paternity has been maintained by making genetic connection to either the father or the mother the defining feature of kinship, *Recreating Motherhood*, p. 36.
42. Ibid., p. 87f.
43. Ibid., p. 18.

4. Donor Insemination and Responsible Parenting

1. Fyodor Dostoevsky, *The Brothers Karamazov*, trans. Constance Garnett (New York: W. W. Norton, 1976), pp. 704–5.
2. See, for example, the responses by Sue Martin, Elizabeth Noble, and James Tunstead Burtchaell to an earlier draft of this chapter published in *Second Opinion*. Their responses appear in *Second Opinion* 17/3 (1992): 95–107.
3. Kass, *Toward a More Natural Science*, p. 74; emphasis added.
4. Ibid., p. 110.
5. And presumably one goal is to raise a healthy, happy child. So how DI might affect the child will be our consideration here.
6. Kass makes this point in connection to IVF, but it is equally true of DI.
7. Kass, *Toward a More Natural Science*, p. 110.
8. *Reproductive Ethics* (Englewood Cliffs, NJ: Prentice-Hall, 1984). Bayles argues that the desire simply to beget children is irrational. Unfortunately, his discussion focuses merely on the abstract desire to beget a child, not on the particular desire to beget a child with a specific person. This latter desire may be perfectly rational, and I have tried to account for this by distinguishing four types of procreative desires, rather than three.
9. This separation may not be so uncommon when we consider cases of uncertain paternity where a woman allows her partner to believe he was the father of the child. Here genetic and social parenthood would be unknowingly separated for the father, but this is not the sort of case I had in mind.
10. Barbara Mays died when Kimberly was two years old.
11. On this point, see Barbara Andolsen, "Recent Works on Reproductive Technology," *Religious Studies Review* 15/3 (July 1989): 213–18.
12. Again, let me emphasize that this is not to say that the intention and the act of creating life are unimportant. In my view they are important. They are just not as important as a commitment to care.
13. See Rothman, *Recreating Motherhood*, p. 127; and Margaret Radin, "Market-Inalienability," *Harvard Law Review* 100/8 (1987): 1849–1937, at 1931.
14. For discussion of a similar view of parenthood, see New Jersey Bioethics Commission Task Force on New Reproductive Practices, "The Lessons of AID for the Family and for Policy on Surrogacy," 1988 (available from the commission).
15. Lisa Sowle Cahill, "The Ethics of Surrogate Motherhood: Biology, Freedom, and Moral Obligation," *Law, Medicine, and Health Care* 16/1–2 (Spring 1988); 69; emphasis added.

16. Ibid., p. 69.

17. Ibid., p. 65.

18. James Tunstead Burtchaell, "The Manufactured Child," *Second Opinion* 17/3 (1992): 104–5.

19. Ibid., p. 104.

20. For an account that appears to imply this view, see Sidney Callahan, "The Ethical Challenge of the New Reproductive Technology," in *Medical Ethics: A Guide for Health Professionals*, ed. John F. Monagle and David C. Thomasma (Rockville, MD: Aspen, 1988), pp. 26–37.

21. Cahill, "The Ethics of Surrogate Motherhood," p. 65.

22. See, e.g., R. Snowden and G. D. Mitchell, *The Artificial Family* (London: Allen and Unwin, 1981).

23. *Artificial Insemination Practice in the United States*, p. 10.

24. They would, however, be sanctioning secrecy, in my view, if they withheld nonidentifying information about donors.

25. As quoted in Ken R. Daniels, "Artificial Insemination Using Donor Semen and the Issue of Secrecy: The Views of Donors and Recipient Couples," *Social Science and Medicine* 27/4 (1988): 379.

26. We can see how the absence of record-keeping can serve to support secrecy by noting that one justification for not telling a child about his or her conception could well be that, in the absence of available records, such information could not be put to any use by the child. He could not seek out his biological father, nor could he even obtain useful medical information.

27. Daniels, "Artificial Insemination Using Donor Semen," p. 378.

28. George J. Annas, "Fathers Anonymous: Beyond the Best Interests of the Sperm Donor," *Family Law Quarterly* 14 (1980): 1–13.

29. Annette Baran and Reuben Pannor, *Lethal Secrets: The Shocking Consequences and Unsolved Problems of Artificial Insemination* (New York: Warner Books, 1989), p. 50.

30. See Daniels, "Artificial Insemination Using Donor Semen," p. 378.

31. Although I would resist using the language of "rights" here, I believe that children conceived through DI should be able to learn the identity of their genetic parents, if they so choose.

32. Sisela Bok, *Lying: Moral Choice in Public and Private Life* (New York: Vintage Books, 1978), p. 224.

33. Baran and Pannor, *Lethal Secrets*, p. 51.

34. Ibid., p. 153.

35. It is worth noting that the first reported court case in an English-speaking jurisdiction that considered the issue of donor insemination and adultery defined adultery as follows: "The essence of the offense of adultery consists, not in the moral turpitude of the act of sexual intercourse, but in the voluntary surrender to another person of the reproductive powers or faculties of the guilty person; and any submission of those powers to the service of enjoyment of any person other than the husband or the wife comes with the definition of 'adultery.' " As quoted in Carmel Shalev, *Birth Power: The Case for Surrogacy* (New Haven: Yale University Press, 1989), p. 22.

36. Burtchael, "The Manufactured Child," p. 105.

37. *Instruction*, p. 23.

38. Ibid., p. 24.

39. Ibid.

40. Kass, *Toward a More Natural Science*, p. 109.

41. *Instruction*, p. 23; Kass, *Toward a More Natural Science*, p. 113.

42. Jarrett Richardson, "The Role of a Psychiatric Consultant to an Artificial Insemination Donor Program," *Psychiatric Annals* 17/2 (1987): 101–5, at 102.

43. For a review of this literature, see Herbert Waltzer, "Psychological and Legal Aspects of Artificial Insemination (AID): An Overview," *American Journal of Psychotherapy*, 36/1 (1982): 91–102.

44. On this point see H. J. Sants, "Genealogical Bewilderment in Children with Substitute Parents," *British Journal of Medical Psychology* 37 (1964): 133–41.

45. Michael Humphrey, "A Fresh Look at Genealogical Bewilderment," *British Journal of Medical Psychology* 59/2 (1986): 133–40.

46. See, for example, Lionel Hersov, "Aspects of Adoption," *Journal of Child Psychology and Psychiatry and Allied Disciplines* 31/4 (1990): 503, and David Brodzinsky, "Adjustment to Adoption," *Clinical Psychology Review* 7 (1987): 29.

47. Baran and Pannor, *Lethal Secrets*, p. 152. See also Marie Meggitt, "Humanizing Community Adoption and Donor Conception Practices," in *Proceedings of the Conference on Adoption and AID: Access to Information*, ed. Anna-Marie Cushan (Monash Centre for Human Bioethics, Melbourne, 1983).

48. I want to emphasize that when I talk about being "forced to choose," I am referring to cases like that of Kimberly Mays, where choice is in some way inescapable. I am not suggesting that infertile couples deciding about DI are forced to choose between genetic and social parenthood. Much of James Burtchaell's response to an earlier version of my argument was based on this misreading and was consequently misdirected.

49. For a fine discussion of the social practice of parenting, see Sara Ruddick, *Maternal Thinking: Toward a Politics of Peace* (Boston: Beacon Press, 1989).

50. On this point, see also Robertson's essay "Technology and Motherhood."

51. There is, however, a second way in which IVF with donor eggs is significantly different from DI, and this difference makes IVF with donor eggs more worrisome than DI. In the case of DI, there is no risk in donating. In clinics with a careful screening program, donating sperm may be time-consuming and somewhat inconvenient, but the procedure for recovering sperm is obviously noninvasive and free of danger. The same cannot be said of donating eggs. As with most IVF procedures, donating eggs will require hormone stimulation of ovulation and surgical removal of eggs. I have discussed the risks associated with these procedures in chapter 2. The difference in this case is that the woman undertaking these risks is not seeking to overcome her own infertility. We must thus ask why a woman would be willing to take such risks. Since egg donors are paid for their "time," one likely and disturbing answer is that egg donors take the risks because they need the money.

5. Parenting for Profit

1. Shabir Bhimji, "Womb for Rent: Ethical Aspects of Surrogate Motherhood," *Canadian Medical Association Journal* 137/12 (1987): 1132–35, at 1132.

2. *Surrogate Parenting v. Kentucky* 704 S.W. 2d 209 (KY 1986).

3. Peter Bowal, "Surrogate Procreation: A Motherhood Issue in Legal Obscurity," *Queen's Law Quarterly* 9/1 (1983): 13.

4. Carmel Shalev, *Birth Power: The Case for Surrogacy*, p. 87.

5. *Surrogate Parenting v. Kentucky* 704 S.W. 2d 212 (KY 1986).

6. *In Re Baby M* 525 A. 2d 1165 (NJ Superior Court 1987).

7. For a useful discussion of equal protection laws as applied to surrogacy, see Alexander M. Capron and Margaret J. Radin, "Choosing Family Law over Contract Law as a Paradigm for Surrogate Motherhood," *Law, Medicine and Health Care* 16/1–2 (Spring 1988): 38f.

8. *In Re Baby M* 1128, 1165. Judge Sorkow was quoting from an earlier Supreme Court decision, *Reed v. Reed* 404 U.S. 71, 76.

9. *In the Matter of Baby M* 537 A. 2d 1227 (NJ 1988), 1254. The court also disputed the Sterns' claim that the sperm donor section of the New Jersey Parentage Act implies a legislative policy that favors surrogacy. In the court's words, "The Parentage Act's silence, however, with respect to surrogacy, rather than supporting, defeats any contention that surrogacy should receive treatment parallel to the sperm donor artificial insemination situation" (p. 1250).

10. Ibid., p. 1249.

11. Lori Andrews, "Surrogate Motherhood: The Challenge for Feminists," *Law, Medicine and Health Care* 16/1–2 (Spring 1988): 78.

12. On the standards for gender classifications, see Rotunda, Nowak, and Young, *Treatise on Constitutional Law: Substance and Procedure,* sections 18.20 to 18.24.

13. Andrews, "Surrogate Motherhood," p. 78.

14. *International Union, United Automobile, Aerospace and Agricultural Implement Workers of America, UAW, et al. v. Johnson Controls* 111 S. Ct. 1196. The Supreme Court ruled that fetal protection policies of Johnson Controls barring fertile women from jobs involving potentially dangerous lead exposure was a violation of Title VII of the Civil Rights Act of 1964.

15. For a discussion of assessing men's responsibilities to fetuses, see Thomas H. Murray, "Moral Obligations to the Not-Yet Born: The Fetus as Patient," *Ethical and Legal Issues in Perinatology* 14/2 (June 1987): 329–43.

16. *In Re Baby M* 1164.

17. Ruth Macklin, "Is There Anything Wrong with Surrogate Motherhood? An Ethical Analysis," *Law, Medicine and Health Care* 16/1–2 (Spring 1988): 60.

18. Larry Gostin, "A Civil Liberties Analysis of Surrogacy Arrangements," *Law, Medicine and Health Care* 16/1–2 (Spring 1988): 14.

19. George J. Annas, "Fairy Tales Surrogate Mothers Tell," *Law, Medicine and Health Care* 16/1–2 (Spring 1988): 31.

20. Rothman, *Recreating Motherhood,* p. 20.

21. Ibid., p. 238.

22. Radin, "Market Inalienability," p. 1880.

23. As quoted by Radin, ibid., p. 1863.

24. Ibid., p. 1880–81.

25. Thanks to Richard B. Miller for pointing this out to me.

26. David H. Smith, "Wombs for Rent, Selves for Sale? *Journal of Contemporary Health Law and Policy* 4 (1988): 23–36, at 31.

27. Annas, "Fairy Tales Surrogate Mothers Tell," p. 28.

28. I am not here talking about short-term pregnancies, but pregnancies where a woman carries the developing child to birth.

29. On this point, see Lisa Sowle Cahill, "Ethics of Surrogate Motherhood," p. 66.

30. Nel Noddings, *Caring: A Feminine Approach to Ethics and Moral Education* (Berkeley: University of California Press, 1984).

6. The Myth and Reality of Current Adoption Practice

1. David N. James, "Artificial Insemination: A Reexamination," *Philosophy and Theology* 2 (Summer 1988): 305–26.

2. Ibid., p. 315.

3. Ibid., p. 316.

4. See Hersov, "Aspects of Adoption."

5. U.S. Department of Commerce, Bureau of Census. *Statistical Abstract of United States,* 110th ed., 1990, p. 370.

6. National Committee for Adoption, *1989 Adoption Factbook* (Washington, 1989), p. 207.

7. I say "strictly speaking" because some states require adoption intermediaries to obtain licenses, at which point they are considered agencies, although adoptions arranged by these "agencies" are still obviously independent adoptions.

8. *Adoption Factbook*, p. 207.

9. Although there may be no home study before placement of the child, all states require a home study before finalization of the adoption. See William Meezan, Sanford Katz, and Eva Manoff Russo, *Adoptions without Agencies: A Study of Independent Adoptions* (New York: Child Welfare League of America, 1978).

10. *Adoption Factbook*, p. 170.

11. Ibid., pp. 121–22.

12. Ibid., p. 20.

13. Ibid., pp. 101–103.

14. Eva Y. Deykin, Lee Campbell, and Patricia Patti, "The Postadoption Experience of Surrendering Parents," *American Journal of Orthopsychiatry* 54 (2) (April 1984): 273.

15. Edward K. Rynearson, "Relinquishment and Its Maternal Complications: A Preliminary Study," *American Journal of Psychiatry* 139 (1982): 339.

16. George M. Burnell and Mary Ann Norfleet, "Women Who Place Their Infant Up for Adoption: A Pilot Study," *Patient Counseling and Health Education* (Summer/Fall 1979): 169.

17. For an endorsement of such a strategy to increase the number of domestic adoptions, see Charlotte Low Allen, "Special Delivery: Overcoming the Barriers to Adoption," *Policy Review* (Summer 1989): 46–53.

18. For a description of the fate of homeless women and children in New York City, see Jonathan Kozol's *Rachel and Her Children* (New York: Fawcett Columbine, 1988).

19. Ibid., p. 49.

20. Ibid., p. 48.

21. Robin Winkler and Margaret van Keppel, *Relinquishing Mothers in Adoption*, Melbourne: Institute of Family Studies Monograph #3, 1984, p. 1.

22. Rothman, *Recreating Motherhood*, p. 126.

23. Ibid., p. 130.

24. Margaret Howard, "Transracial Adoption: Analysis of the Best Interests Standard," *Notre Dame Law Review* 59 (1984): 503–55. See also Elizabeth Bartholet, "Where Do Black Children Belong? The Politics of Race Matching in Adoption," *University of Pennsylvania Law Review* 139 (May 1991): 1163–1256.

25. Howard, "Transracial Adoption," pp. 516–18

26. As quoted in Bartholet, p. 1190.

27. I agree with Bartholet that the answer is complex and probably involves a combination of white racism, black nationalism, and an unquestioned commitment to making adoption as close to biological kinship as possible.

28. Howard, "Transracial Adoption," p. 518.

29. Ibid., p. 517. Bartholet points out that the position of the NABSW on transracial adoption has not changed.

30. Ibid., p. 535.

31. Ibid., p. 540. See also the studies cited in Owen Gill and Barbara Jackson, *Adoption and Race* (New York: St. Martin's Press, 1983).

32. Bartholet, p. 1183.

BIBLIOGRAPHY

Allen, Anita L. *Uneasy Access: Privacy for Women in a Free Society.* Totowa, NJ: Rowman and Littlefield, 1988.

Allen, Charlotte Low. "Special Delivery: Overcoming the Barriers to Adoption." *Policy Review* (Summer 1989): 46–53.

American Academy of Pediatrics. Committee on Adoptions. "Identity Development in Adopted Children." *Pediatrics* 47/5 (May 1971): 948–49.

American College of Obstetricians and Gynecologists. Committee on Ethics. "Ethical Issues in Human In Vitro Fertilization and Embryo Placement." *ACOG Committee Statement.* July 1986. Washington, D.C.

American Fertility Society. Ethics Committee. "Ethical Considerations of the New Reproductive Technologies." *Fertility and Sterility* Supplement 46/3 (September 1986): v.-94s.

———. (1986–87). "Ethical Considerations of the New Reproductive Technologies in Light of 'Instruction on the Respect for Human Life in Its Origin and on Dignity of Procreation.'" *Fertility and Sterility* 49/2 (February 1988): i-7S.

Amnon, David, and Dalia Avidan. "Artificial Insemination Donor: Clinical and Psychologic Aspects." *Fertility and Sterility* 27/5 (May 1976): 528–32.

Anderson, W. French. "Prospects for Human Gene Therapy." *Science* 226 (October 26, 1984): 401–9.

Andolsen, Barbara. "Recent Works on Reproductive Technology." *Religious Studies Review* 15/3 (July 1989): 213–18.

Andrews, Lori B. "The Aftermath of Baby M: Proposed State Laws on Surrogate Motherhood." *Hastings Center Report* (October/November 1987): 31–40.

———. *Between Strangers: Surrogate Mothers, Expectant Fathers, and Brave New Babies.* New York: Harper and Row, 1989.

———. "Brave New Baby." *Student Lawyer* (December 1983): 25–29, 46f.

———. "Ethical Aspects of In-Vitro Fertilization and Artificial Insemination by Donor." *Urologic Clinics of North America* 14/3 (August 1987): 633–42.

———. "Legal and Ethical Aspects of New Reproductive Technologies." *Clinical Obstetrics and Gynecology* 29/1 (March 1986): 190–204.

———. "The Legal Status of the Embryo." *Loyola Law Review* 32 (1986): 357–409.

———. "The Stork Market: Legal Regulation of the New Reproductive Technologies." *Whittier Law Review* 6 (1984): 789–98.

———. "Surrogate Motherhood: The Challenge for Feminists." *Law, Medicine and Health Care* 16/1-2 (Spring 1988): 72–80.

———. "When Baby's Mother Is Also Grandma and Sister." *Hastings Center Report* (October 1985): 29–31.

Annas, George J. "Fairy Tales Surrogate Mothers Tell." *Law, Medicine and Health Care* 16/1-2 (Spring 1988): 27–33.

———. "Fathers Anonymous: Beyond the Best Interests of the Sperm Donor." *Family Law Quarterly* 14 (1980): 1–13.

———. "The Impact of Medical Technology on the Pregnant Woman's Right to Privacy." *American Journal of Law and Medicine* 13/2–3 (1987): 213–32.

———. "Making Babies without Sex." *American Journal of Public Health* 74/12 (December 1984): 1415–17.

———. "Prefatory Prediction and Mindless Mimicry: The Case of Mary O'Connor." *Hastings Center Report* (December 1988): 31–33.

————. "Redefining Parenthood and Protecting Embryos: Why We Need New Laws." *Hastings Center Report* (October 1984): 50–52.

Annas, George J., and Sherman Elias. "In Vitro Fertilization and Embryo Transfer: Medicolegal Aspects of a New Technique to Create a Family." *Family Law Quarterly* 17/2 (Summer 1983): 199–223.

Arditti, Rita, Duelli Klein Renate, and Shelley Minden, eds. *Test-Tube Women: What Future for Motherhood?* London: Pandora Press, 1984.

Atwell, Barbara. "Surrogacy and Adoption: A Case of Incompatibility." *Columbia Human Rights Law Review* 20/1 (1988): 1–59.

Australia. Victoria. Committee to Consider the Social, Ethical and Legal Issues Arising from In Vitro Fertilization. *Interim Report.* September 1982.

————. *Issues Paper on Donor Gametes in IVF.* April 1983.

————. *Report on Donor Gametes in IVF.* August 1983.

————. *Report on the Disposition of Embryos Produced by In Vitro Fertilization.* August 1984.

Baran, Annette, and Reuben Pannor. *Lethal Secrets: The Shocking Consequences and Unsolved Problems of Artificial Insemination.* New York: Warner Books, 1989.

Barnet, Robert. "Surrogate Parenting: Social, Legal and Ethical Implications." *Linacre Quarterly* 54/3 (August 1987): 28–38.

Bartholet, Elizabeth. "Where Do Black Children Belong? The Politics of Race Matching in Adoption." *University of Pennsylvania Law Review* 139 (May 1991): 1163–1256.

Baruch, Elaine Hoffman, Amadeo F. D'Amado, Jr., and Joni Seager, eds. *Embryos, Ethics and Women's Rights: Exploring the New Reproductive Technologies.* New York: Harrington Press, 1988.

Bayles, Michael D. *Reproductive Ethics.* Englewood Cliffs, NJ: Prentice-Hall, 1984.

Bell, Susan, et al. "Reclaiming Reproductive Control: A Feminist Approach to Fertility Consciousness." *Science for the People* 12 (January/February 1980): 6–9, 30–35.

Benet, Mary Kathleen. *The Politics of Adoption.* New York: Free Press, 1976.

Berger, David M., Abraham Eisen, Jack Shuber, and Kenneth F. Doody. "Psychological Patterns in Donor Insemination Couples." *Canadian Journal of Psychiatry* 31/9 (December 1986): 818–23.

Berkowitz, Richard L., et al. "Selective Reduction of Multifetal Pregnancies in the First Trimester." *New England Journal of Medicine* 318/16 (April 21, 1988): 1043–47.

Bezanson, Randall P. "Solomon Would Weep: A Comment on 'In the Matter of Baby M' and the Limits of Judicial Authority." *Law, Medicine and Health Care* 16/1–2 (Spring 1988): 126–30.

Bhimji, Shabir. "Womb for Rent: Ethical Aspects of Surrogate Motherhood." *Canadian Medical Association Journal* 137/12 (1987): 1132–35.

Bigelow, John, and Robert Pargetter. "Morality, Potential Persons and Abortion." *American Philosophical Quarterly* 25/2 (April 1988): 173–81.

Birnstiel, Max L., and Meinrad Busslinger. "Dangerous Liaisons: Spermatozoa as Natural Vectors for Foreign DNA?" *Cell* 57/5 (June 2, 1989): 701–702.

Blakely, Mary Kay. "Surrogate Mothers: For Whom Are They Working?" *Ms.* (March 1983): 18–20.

Blank, Robert H. *Redefining Human Life: Reproductive Technologies and Social Policy.* Boulder, CO: Westview Press, 1984.

Blustein, Jeffrey. *Parents and Children.* New York: Oxford University Press, 1982.

Bodmer, Walter F. "The William Allan Memorial Award Address: Gene Clusters, Genome Organization, and Complex Phenotypes. When the Sequence Is Known, What Will It Mean?" *American Journal of Human Genetics* 33 (1981): 664–82.

Bok, Sisela. *Lying: Moral Choice in Public and Private Life.* New York: Vintage Books, 1979.

Bonnicksen, Andrea L. "Embryo Freezing: Ethical Issues in the Clinical Setting." *Hastings Center Report* (December 1988): 26–30.

———. "Feminist Dimensions of In Vitro Fertilization." *Biolaw* 2/2 (August 1986): S:31–S:36.

Boswell, John. *The Kindness of Strangers.* New York: Pantheon Books, 1988.

Bowal, Peter. "Surrogate Procreation: A Motherhood Issue in Legal Obscurity." *Queen's Law Journal* 9/1 (Fall 1983): 5–34.

Boyle, Joseph. "An Introduction to the Vatican Instruction on Reproductive Technologies." *Linacre Quarterly* 55/1 (February 1988): 20–28.

Brahams, Diana. "The Hasty British Ban on Commercial Surrogacy." *Hastings Center Report* 17/1 (February 1987): 16–19.

Brodzinsky, David M. "Adjustment to Adoption: A Psychosocial Perspective." *Clinical Psychology Review* 7 (1987): 25–47.

Brodzinsky, David M., Carol Radice, Loreen Huffman, and Karen Merkler. "Prevalence of Clinically Significant Symptomatology in a Nonclinical Sample of Adopted and Nonadopted Children." *Journal of Clinical Child Psychology* 16/4 (1987): 350–56.

Burke, Carolyn. "The Adult Adoptee's Constitutional Right to Know His Origins." *Southern California Law Reveiw* 48 (1975): 1196–1220.

Burnell, George M., and Mary Ann Norfleet. "Women Who Place Their Infant Up for Adoption: A Pilot Study." *Patient Counseling and Health Education* (Summer/Fall 1979): 169–72.

Burtchaell, James Tunstead. "The Manufactured Child." *Second Opinion* 17/3 (1992): 104–5.

Caffara, Msgr. Carlo. "The Moral Problem of Artificial Insemination." *Linacre Quarterly* 55/1 (February 1988): 37–43.

Cahill, Lisa Sowle. *Between the Sexes: Foundations for a Christian Ethics of Sexuality.* Philadelphia: Fortress Press, 1985.

———. "The Ethics of Surrogate Motherhood: Biology, Freedom and Moral Obligation." *Law, Medicine and Health Care* 16/1–2 (Spring 1988): 65–71.

———. "The 'Seamless Garment': Life in Its Beginnings." *Theological Studies* 46/1 (March 1985): 64–80.

———. "Women, Marriage, Parenthood: What Are Their 'Natures'?" *Logos* 9 (1988): 11–35.

Cahill, Lisa Sowle, and Richard A. McCormick. "The Vatican Document on Bioethics: Two Responses." *America* (March 28, 1987): 246–48.

Callahan, Sidney C. "The Ethical Challenge of the New Reproductive Technology." in *Medical Ethics: A Guide for Health Professionals,* ed. John F. Monagle and David C. Thomasma. Rockville: Aspen, 1988.

———. *In Good Conscience: Reason and Emotion in Moral Decision Making.* San Francisco: Harper and Row, 1991.

———. "The Role of Emotions in Ethical Decisionmaking." *Hastings Center Report* 18/3 (1988): 9–14.

Caplan, Arthur L. "The Ethics of In Vitro Fertilization." *Primary Care* 13/2 (June 1986): 241–53.

———. "Should Foetuses or Infants Be Utilized as Organ Donors?" *Bioethics* 1/2 (1987): 119–40.

Caplan, Arthur L., H. Tristram Engelhardt, Jr., and James J. McCartney, eds. *Concepts of Health and Disease: Interdisciplinary Perspectives.* London: Addison-Wesley, 1981.

Capron, Alexander M. "Bioethics on the Congressional Agenda." *Hastings Center Report* (March/April 1989): 22–23.

Capron, Alexander M., and Margaret J. Radin. "Choosing Family Law over Contract Law as a Paradigm for Surrogate Motherhood." *Law, Medicine and Health Care* 16/1–2 (Spring 1988): 34–43.

Carney, Brian J. "Where Do the Children Go?: Surrogate Mother Contracts and the Best Interests of the Child." *Suffolk University Law Review* 22 (1988): 1187–1217.

Caskey, C. Thomas. "Genetic Therapy: Somatic Gene Transplants." *Hospital Practice* 8 (August 15, 1987): 181–98.

Chalmers, D. R. C. "No Primrose Path: Surrogacy and the Role of Criminal Law." *Medicine and Law* 7/6 (1989): 595–606.

Chapman, David E. "Retailing Human Organs under the Uniform Commercial Code." *John Marshall Law Review* 16 (1983): 393–417.

Chapman, Fern Schumer. "Going for Gold in the Baby Business." *Fortune* (September 17, 1984): 41–47.

Charney, Mitchell A. "The Rebirth of Private Adoptions." *ABA Journal* 71 (June 1985): 52–55.

Charo, R. Alta. *Artificial Insemination Practice in the United States: Summary of a 1987 Survey.* U.S. Congress. Office of Technology Assessment. August 9, 1988.

———. "Legislative Approaches to Surrogate Motherhood." *Law, Medicine and Health Care* 16/1–2 (Spring 1988): 96–112.

———. Problems in Commercialized Surrogate Mothering." *Women & Health* 13/1–2 (1987): 195–201.

Chell, Byron. "But Murderers Can Have All the Children They Want: Surrogacy and Public Policy." *Theoretical Medicine* 9 (1988): 3–21.

Christiaens, Marc. "Artificial Insemination by Donor and the View of Man." *European Journal of Obstetrics and Gynecology and Reproductive Biology* 28 (1988): 347–52.

Clamar, Aphrodite. "Artificial Insemination by Donor: The Anonymous Pregnancy." *American Journal of Forensic Psychology* 2/1 (1984): 27–37.

Clapp, Marilyn J. "State Prohibition of Fetal Experimentation and the Fundamental Right of Privacy." *Columbia Law Review* 88/5 (June 1988): 1073–97.

Cohen, Sherrill, and Nadine Taub, eds. *Reproductive Laws for the 1990s.* Clifton, NJ: Humana Press, 1989.

Congregation for the Doctrine of the Faith. *Instruction on Respect for Human Life in Its Origin and on the Dignity of Procreation: Replies to Certain Questions of the Day.* Washington: United States Catholic Conference, Publication No. 156–3, 1987.

Conover, J. C., and R. B. L. Gwatkin. "Fertilization of Zona-drilled Mouse Oocytes Treated with a Monoclonal Antibody to the Zona Glycoprotein, ZP3." *Journal of Experimental Zoology* 247/1 (1988): 113–18.

Corea, Gena. *The Mother Machine: Reproductive Technologies from Artificial Insemination to Artificial Wombs.* New York: Harper and Row, 1985.

———. "Unnatural Selection: The Menace of High-Tech Motherhood." *The Progressive* (January 1986): 22–24.

Corea, Gena, et al. *Man-Made Women: How New Reproductive Technologies Affect Women.* Bloomington: Indiana University Press, 1987.

Coughlan, Michael J. *The Vatican, the Law and the Human Embryo.* Iowa City: University of Iowa Press, 1990.

Council for Science and Society. *Human Procreation: Ethical Aspects of the New Techniques.* Oxford: Oxford University Press, 1984.

Crowe, Christine. "'Women Want It': In-Vitro Fertilization and Women's Motivations for Participation." *Women's Studies International Forum* 8/6 (1985): 547–52.

Culliton, Barbara J. "Gene Therapy Guidelines Revised." *Science* 228 (May 3, 1985): 561–62.

———. "Gene Therapy: Research in Public." *Science* 227 (February 1, 1985): 493–96.

------. "NIH Asked to Tighten Gene Therapy Rules." *Science* 233 (September 26, 1986): 1378–79.

Curtis, Carolyn. "The Psychological Parent Doctrine in Custody Disputes between Foster Parents and Biological Parents." *Columbia Journal of Law and Social Problems* 16 (1980): 149–92.

D'Adamo, Amadeo F., Jr., and Elaine Hoffman Baruch. "Whither the Womb? Myths, Machines and Mothers." *Frontiers* 9/1 (1986): 72–79.

Dale, Michael J. "The Burger Court and Issues of Illegitimacy: A Brief Overlook." *Children's Legal Rights Journal* 9/1 (Winter 1988): 9–15.

Daniels, Ken R. "Artificial Insemination Using Donor Semen and the Issue of Secrecy: The Views of Donors and Recipient Couples." *Social Science and Medicine* 27/4 (1988): 377–83.

------. "Psychosocial Issues Associated with Being a Semen Donor." *Clinical Reproduction and Fertility* 4/5 (October 1986): 341–51.

Daniels, Norman. "Reflective Equilibrium and Archimedean Points." *Canadian Journal of Philosophy* 10/1 (March 1980): 83–103.

------. "Wide Reflective Equilibrium and Theory Acceptance in Ethics." *Journal of Philosophy* 76 (1979): 256–82.

Danis, Mark W. "Fetal Tissue Transplants: Restricting Recipient Designation." *Hastings Law Journal* 39/5 (July 1988): 1079–1107.

Davis, Joseph H., and Dirck W. Brown. "Artificial Insemination by Donor (AID) and the Use of Surrogate Mothers: Social and Psychological Impact." *Western Journal of Medicine* 141/1 (July 1984): 127–30.

Davis, Nancy Ann. "Reproductive Technologies and Our Attitudes towards Children." *Logos* 9 (1988): 51–77.

De Cruz, S. P. "Surrogacy, Adoption and Custody: A Case-Study." *Family Law* 18 (March 1988): 100–107.

De Parseval, Genevieve Delaisi, and Anne Fagot-Largeault. "The Status of Artificially Procreated Children: International Disparities." *Bioethics* 2/2 (1988): 136–50.

Depypere, H. T., et al. "Comparison of Zona Cutting and Zona Drilling as Techniques for Assisted Fertilization in the Mouse." *Journal of Reproduction & Fertility* 84/1 (1988): 205–11.

Detering, Klaus. "Phase III Evaluation of Fertility-regulating Agents as Viewed by the Industry." *Human Reproduction* 2/2 (1987): 163–68.

Deykin, Eva Y., Lee Campbell, and Patricia Patti. "The Postadoption Experience of Surrendering Parents." *American Journal of Orthopsychiatry* 54/2 (April 1984): 271–80.

Diamond, Irene, ed. *Families, Politics and Public Policy: A Feminist Dialogue on Women and the State.* New York: Longman, 1983.

Dickson, David. "'Dangerous' Liaisons in Cell Biology." *Science* 244 (June 30, 1989): 1539–40.

Direcks, Anita. "Has the Lesson Been Learned? The DES Story and IVF." In *Made to Order,* ed. Patricia Spallone and Deborah Lynn Steinberg. Oxford: Pergamon Press, 1987.

Donchin, Anne. "The Future of Mothering: Reproductive Technology and Feminist Theory." *Hypatia* 1/2 (Fall 1986): 121–37.

------. "Reproductive Technology and Moral Responsibility: Redefining Parenthood." *The Tasks of Contemporary Philosophy* 12/1 (1986): 265–67.

Donovan, Patricia. "New Reproductive Technologies: Some Legal Dilemmas." *Family Planning Perspectives* 18/2 (March/April 1986): 57–60.

Drori, M. "Reflections on the Effect of Modern Techniques of Fertility on Family Law." *Medicine and Law* 1 (1982): 15–28.

Dworkin, Gerald. "Is More Choice Better than Less?" In *Social and Political Philoso-*

phy, ed. Peter A. French, Jr., Theodore E. Uehling, and Howard K. Welt-stein. Midwest Studies in Philosophy, vol. 7. Minneapolis: University of Minnesota Press, 1982.

Edwards, Robert. *Life before Birth: Reflections on the Embryo Debate.* New York: Basic Books, 1989.

Elias, Sherman, and George J. Annas. "Social Policy Considerations in Noncoital Reproduction." *Journal of the American Medical Association* 255/1 (January 3, 1986): 62–68.

Elshtain, Jean Bethke. "Technology as Destiny: The New Eugenics Challenges Feminism." *The Progressive* (June 1989): 19–23.

Ely, John Hart. "The Wages of Crying Wolf: A Comment on *Roe v. Wade.*" *Yale Law Review* 82 (1973): 1920–49.

Engelhardt, H. Tristram, Jr. *The Foundations of Bioethics.* New York: Oxford University Press, 1986.

———. "Persons and Humans: Refashioning Ourselves in a Better Image and Likeness." *Zygon* 19/3 (September 1984): 281–95.

Feinberg, Joel. "Comment: Wrongful Conception and the Right Not to Be Harmed." *Harvard Journal of Law and Public Policy* 8/1 (1985): 57–77.

Feinerman, James V. "A Comparative Look at Surrogacy." *Georgetown Law Journal* 76 (1988): 1837–44.

Figueira-McDonough, Josefina, and Rosemary Sarri, eds. *The Trapped Woman: Catch-22 in Deviance and Control.* Sage Sourcebooks for the Human Services Series. Newbury Park: Sage, 1987.

Firestone, Shulamith. *The Dialectic of Sex.* New York: Morrow, 1970.

Fishel, Simon. "Assisted Human Reproduction and Embryonic Surgery: The Ethical Issues." *Annals of the New York Academy of Sciences* 530 (1988): 54–72.

Fleming, John I. "A Critical Evaluation of the Vatican's Instruction on Respect for Human Life." *Linacre Quarterly* 55/1 (February 1988): 13–19.

Fletcher, John C. "Moral Problems and Ethical Issues in Prospective Human Gene Therapy." *Virginia Law Review* 69/1 (February 1983): 515–46.

Fletcher, John C., and Mark I. Evans. "Maternal Bonding in Early Fetal Ultrasound Examinations." *New England Journal of Medicine* 308 (February 17, 1983): 392–93.

Fletcher, John C., and Kenneth J. Ryan. "Federal Regulations for Fetal Research: A Case for Reform." *Law, Medicine and Health Care* 15/3 (Fall 1987): 126–38.

Fletcher, Joseph. *Morals and Medicine: The Moral Problems of the Patient's Right to Know the Truth, Contraception, Artificial Insemination, Sterilization, Euthanasia.* Princeton: Princeton University Press, 1954.

Flynn, Eileen P. *Human Fertilization In Vitro: A Catholic Moral Perspective.* Lanham, MD: University Press of America, 1984.

Fox, Jeffrey L. "Nonsurgical Ovum Transfer." *High Technology* 7/6 (June 1987): 13–14.

Francis, Gail R., and Janet A. Nosek. "Ethical Considerations in Contemporary Reproductive Technologies." *Journal of Perinatal and Neonatal Nursing* 1/3 (January 1988): 37–48.

Frankfurt, Harry G. *The Importance of What We Care About: Philosophical Essays.* Cambridge: Cambridge University Press, 1988.

Fredericks, Christopher M., John D. Paulson, and Alan H. DeCherney, eds. *Foundations of In Vitro Fertilization.* Washington, DC: Hemisphere, 1987.

Freedman, Benjamin, Patrick J. Taylor, Thomas Wonnacott, and Stanley Brown. "Non-medical Selection Criteria for Artificial Insemination and Adoption." *Clinical Reproduction and Fertility* 5 (1987): 55–66.

Friedman, Susan Stanford. "Creativity and the Childbirth Metaphor: Gender Difference in Literary Discourse." *Feminist Studies* 13/1 (Spring 1987): 49–82.

Friedmann, Theodore. "Progress toward Human Gene Therapy." *Science* 244 (June 16, 1989): 1275–80.

Gallagher, Janet. "The Fetus and the Law: Whose Life Is It Anyway?" *Ms.* (September 1984): 62–66, 134–35.

Geller, S. "The Child and/or the Embryo: To Whom Does It Belong?" *Human Reproduction* 1/8 (1986): 56–57.

Gerstel, Gerda. "A Psychoanalytic View of Artificial Donor Insemination." *American Journal of Psychotherapy* 17 (1963): 64–77.

Gill, Owen, and Barbara Jackson. *Adoption and Race.* New York: St. Martin's Press, 1983.

Glendon, Mary Ann. *The New Family and the New Property.* Toronto: Butterworths, 1981.

Gleve, Katherine. "Rethinking Feminist Attitudes towards Motherhood." *Feminist Review* 25 (Spring 1987): 38–45.

Gloor, Carol. "Breaking the Seal: Constitutional and Statutory Approaches to Adult Adoptees' Right to Identity." *Northwestern University Law Review* 75/2 (1980): 316–44.

Gold, Michael. "Adoption: A New Problem for Jewish Law." *Judaism* 36 (Fall 1987): 443–50.

Goldman, Brian. "Infertility Giving Birth to New Problems for Doctors and Lawyers." *Canadian Medical Association Journal* 138/2 (January 15, 1988): 166–67.

Gordon, Jon W., Larry Greenfeld, G. John Garrisi, et al. "Fertilization of Human Oocytes by Sperm from Infertile Males after Zona Pellucida Drilling." *Fertility and Sterility* 50/1 (July 1988): 68–73.

Gostin, Larry. "A Civil Liberties Analysis of Surrogacy Arrangements." *Law, Medicine and Health Care* 16/1–2 (Spring 1988): 7–17.

———. "Forum on Surrogate Motherhood. Introduction." *Law, Medicine and Health Care* 16/1–2 (Spring 1988): 5–6.

———, ed. *Surrogate Motherhood: Politics and Privacy.* Bloomington: Indiana University Press, 1990.

Greco, Paul J. "Parental Guidance Suggested: A Proposal for Regulating Surrogate Parenthood." *Columbia Journal of Law and Social Problems* 22 (1989): 115–80.

Greenfeld, Dorothy, Michael P. Diamond, Ruth L. Breslin, and Alan DeCherney. "Infertility and the New Reproductive Technology: A Role for Social Work." *Social Work in Health Care* 12/2 (Winter 1986): 71–81.

Greer, Germaine. *Sex and Destiny: The Politics of Human Fertility.* New York: Harper and Row.

Greil, Arthur L., Thomas A. Leitko, and Karen L. Porter. "Infertility: His and Hers." *Gender and Society* 2/2 (June 1988): 172–99.

Grey, Thomas. "Eros, Civilization and the Burger Court." *Law and Contemporary Problems* 43/3 (Summer 1980): 83–100.

Grobstein, Clifford, Michael Flower, and John Mendeloff. "External Human Fertilization: An Evaluation of Policy." *Science* 222 (October 14, 1983): 127–33.

———. "Frozen Embryos: Policy Issues." *New England Journal of Medicine* 312/24 (June 13, 1985): 1584–88.

Gudorf, Christine E. "The Power to Create: Sacraments and Men's Need to Birth." *Horizons* 14/2 (1987): 296–309.

Gustafson, James M. "Nature: Its Status in Theological Ethics." *Logos* 3 (1982): 5–23.

Hafen, Bruce C. "The Constitutional Status of Marriage, Kinship, and Sexual Privacy: Balancing the Individual and Social Interests." *Michigan Law Review* 81 (January 1983): 463–574.

Hager, John W. "Artificial Insemination: Some Practical Considerations for Effective Counseling." *North Carolina Law Review* 39 (1961): 217–37.

Handelsman, David J., et al. "Psychological and Attitudinal Profiles in Donors for Artificial Insemination." *Fertility and Sterility* 43/1 (January 1985): 95–101.

Hanmer, Jalna, and Pat Allen. "Reproductive Engineering: The Final Solution?" *Feminist Issues* (Spring 1982): 53–74.

Hanscombe, Gillian. "The Right to Lesbian Parenthood." *Journal of Medical Ethics* 9 (1983): 133–35.

Harris, George W. "Fathers and Fetuses." *Ethics* 96/3 (April 1986): 594–603.

Harrison, Jeffrey L. "Egoism, Altruism, and Market Illusions: The Limits of Law and Economics." *UCLA Law Review* 33 (1986): 1309–63.

Held, Virginia. "Coercion and Coercive Offers." In *Coercion*, ed. J. Roland Pennock and John W. Chapman. Chicago and New York: Atherton, 1972.

Hellegers, Andre E. "Fetal Development." *Theological Studies* 31 (1970): 3–9.

Henifin, Mary Sue. "Women's Health and the New Reproductive Technologies." *Women and Health* 13/1–2 (1987): 1–7.

Hershman, David. "Access before Adoption: The Decision to Terminate." *Family Law* 18 (December 1988): 491–92.

Hersov, Lionel. "Aspects of Adoption." *Journal of Child Psychology* and *Psychiatry and Allied Disciplines* 31/4 (1990): 493–510.

Herz, Elisabeth K. "Infertility and Bioethical Issues of the New Reproductive Technologies." *Psychiatric Clinics of North America* 12/1 (March 1989): 117–31.

Hewitt, Jonathan. "Preconceptional Sex Selection." *British Journal of Hospital Medicine* 37 (February 1987): 151–55.

Hilderbran, Gregory S. "'In Re Baby Girl Eason': Balancing Three Competing Interests in Third Party Adoptions." *Georgia Law Review* 22 (Summer 1988): 1217–44.

Hill, Edward C. "Your Morality or Mine? An Inquiry into the Ethics of Human Reproduction." *American Journal of Obstetrics and Gynecology* 154/6 (June 1986): 1173–80.

Hill, Malcolm. "Payments for Adopted Children: Right or Wrong?" *Journal of Social Policy* 16/4 (October 1987): 461–88.

Hirsh, Harold L. "Surrogate Motherhood: A Womb in Livery." *Legal Medicine* 5 (1986): 165–98.

Holder, Angela Roddy. *Legal Issues in Pediatrics and Adolescent Medicine.* New Haven: Yale University Press, 1985. [2d. ed.]

———. "Selective Termination of Pregnancy." *Hastings Center Report* (February/ March 1988): 21–22.

———. "Surrogate Motherhood and the Best Interests of Children." *Law, Medicine and Health Care* 16/1–2 (Spring 1988): 51–56.

Hollinger, Joan Heifetz. "From Coitus to Commerce: Legal and Social Consequences of Noncoital Reproduction." *Journal of Law Reform* 18/4 (Summer 1985): 866–932.

Howard, Margaret. "Transracial Adoption: Analysis of the Best Interests Standard." *Notre Dame Law Review* 59 (1984): 503–55.

Hull, Richard T., ed. *Ethical Issues in the New Reproductive Technology.* Belmont, CA: Wadsworth, 1990.

Humphrey, Heather, and Michael Humphrey. "Damaged Identity and the Search for Kinship in Adult Adoptees." *British Journal of Medical Psychology* 62/4 (1989): 301–9.

Humphrey, Michael. "A Fresh Look at Genealogical Bewilderment." *British Journal of Medical Psychology* 59/2 (1986): 133–40.

Jaggar, Alison. *Feminist Politics and Human Nature.* Totowa, NJ: Rowman and Allan-
    held, 1983.
James, David N. "Artificial Insemination: A Reexamination." *Philosophy and Theolo-
    gy* 2 (Summer 1988): 305–26.
Johnsen, Dawn. "A New Threat to Pregnant Women's Autonomy." *Hastings Center
    Report* 17/4 (August 1987): 33–40.
Johnson, Sandra H. "The Baby 'M' Decision: Specific Performance of a Contract for
    Specially Manufactured Goods." *Southern Illinois University Law Journal* 11
    (1987): 1339–48.
Jones, D. Gareth. *Brave New People: Ethical Issues at the Commencement of Life.*
    Leicester, England: Inter-Varsity Press, 1984.
Jones, Kathleen B. "Socialist-Feminist Theories of the Family." *Praxis International* 8
    (October 1988): 284–300.
Jonsen, Albert R. "Transplantation of Fetal Tissue: An Ethicist's Viewpoint." *Clini-
    cal Research* 36/3 (April 1988): 215–19.
Karp, Laurence E., and Roger P. Donahue. "Preimplantational Ectogenesis: Science
    and Speculation concerning *In Vitro* Fertilization and Related Procedures."
    Western Journal of Medicine 124/4 (April 1976): 282–98.
Karpel, Mark A. "Family Secrets: 1. Conceptual and Ethical Issues in the Relational
    Context, 2. Ethical and Practical Considerations in Therapeutic Manage-
    ment." *Family Process* 19 (September 1980): 295–306.
Kass, Leon R. *Toward a More Natural Science: Biology and Human Affairs.* New York:
    Free Press, 1985.
Keane, Noel P. "Legal Problems of Surrogate Motherhood." *Southern Illinois Univer-
    sity Law Journal* 2 (1980): 147–69.
Kennedy, Ian, and R. G. Edwards. "A Critique of the Law Commission Report on
    Injuries to Unborn Children and the Proposed Congenital Disabilities (Civil
    Liability) Bill." *Journal of Medical Ethics* 1 (1975): 116–21.
Kern, Patricia A., and Kathleen M. Ridolfi. "The Fourteenth Amendment's Protec-
    tion of a Woman's Right to Be a Single Parent through Artificial Insemination
    by Donor." *Women's Rights Law Reporter* 7/3 (Spring 1982): 251–84.
King, Patricia A. "The Juridical Status of the Fetus: A Proposal for Legal Protection
    of the Unborn." *Michigan Law Review* 77 (August 1979): 1647–87.
Kirby, M. D. "Bioethics of IVF: The State of the Debate." *Journal of Medical Ethics* 1
    (1984): 45–48.
Kleegman, Sophia, et al. "Artificial Donor Insemination." *Medical Aspects of Human
    Sexuality* 5 (1970): 85–111.
Klibanoff, Elton B. "Genealogical Information in Adoption: The Adoptee's Quest
    and the Law." *Family Law Quarterly* 11/2 (Summer 1977): 185–98.
Kolata, Gina. "Fetal Surgery for Neural Defects?" *Science* 221 (July 29, 1983): 441.
———. "First Trimester Prenatal Diagnosis: A New Method of Prenatal Diagnosis
    May Largely Replace Amniocentesis." *Science* 221 (September 9, 1983): 1031–
    32.
———. "Panel Urges Newborn Sickle Cell Screening." *Science* 236 (April 17, 1987):
    259–60.
Kolder, Veronika E. B., Janet Gallagher, and Michael T. Parsons. "Court-ordered
    Obstetrical Interventions." *New England Journal of Medicine* 316/19 (May 7,
    1987): 1192–96.
Kopytoff, Barbara K. "Surrogate Motherhood: Questions of Law and Values."
    University of San Francisco Law Review 22 (Winter/Spring 1988): 205–49.
Koshland, Daniel E., Jr. "Sequencing the Human Genome." *Science* 236 (May 1,
    1987): 505.
Kozol, Jonathan. *Rachel and Her Children: Homeless Families in America.* New York:
    Fawcett Columbine, 1988.

Krauthammer, Charles. "Political Malpractice: The Ban on Fetal Transplantation." *Washington Post* (November 10, 1989): A27.

La Femina, Diana. "The Lawyer's Role in the Independent Adoption Process: Parental Consent and Best Interests of the Child." *Touro Law Review* 3/2 (1987): 283–314.

Lafollette, Hugh. "Licensing Parents." *Philosophy & Public Affairs* 9/2 (1980): 182–97.

Lamport, Ann T. "The Genetics of Secrecy in Adoption, Artificial Insemination, and In Vitro Fertilization." *American Journal of Law and Medicine* 14/1 (1988): 109–24.

Lansner, David J. "A Review of New Legislation Affecting Family Law Practice." *New York Law Journal* 200/57 (September 21, 1988): 1–3.

Lappe, Marc. "The Limits of Genetic Inquiry." *Hastings Center Report* 17/4 (August 1987): 5–10.

La Puma, John, David L. Schiedermayer, and John Grover. "Surrogacy and Shakespeare: The Merchant's Contract Revisited." *American Journal of Obstetrics and Gynecology* 160/1 (January 1989): 59–62.

Lavitrano, Marialuisa, et al. "Sperm Cells as Vectors for Introducing Foreign DNA into Eggs: Genetic Transformation of Mice." *Cell* 57/5 (June 2, 1989): 717–23.

Lawler, Ronald D. "Moral Reflections on the New Technologies: A Catholic Analysis." *Women and Health* 13/1–2 (1987): 167–77.

Lebacqz, Karen, ed. *Genetics, Ethics and Parenthood.* New York: Pilgrim Press, 1983.

Ledley, Fred D. "Somatic Gene Therapy for Human Disease: Background and Prospects." *Journal of Pediatrics* 110/1–2 (January/February 1987): 1–8, 167–74.

Leiberman, J. R., M. Mazor, W. Chaim, and A. Cohen. "The Fetal Right to Live." *Obstetrics and Gynecology* 53/4 (April 1979): 515–17.

Liebard, Odile M., comp., *Love and Sexuality.* Wilmington, NC: Consortium Books, 1978.

Lumley, Judith. "The Proposed Victorian Donor Gamete Register." *Clinical Reproduction and Fertility* 4/1 (February 1986): 39–43.

Lynch, Joseph H. *Godparents and Kinship in Early Medieval Europe.* Princeton: Princeton University Press, 1986.

Lynn, Suzanne M. "Technology and Reproductive Rights: How Advances in Technology Can Be Used to Limit Women's Reproductive Rights." *Women's Rights Law Reporter* 7/3 (Spring 1982): 223–27.

MacCormack, Carol P., ed. *Ethnography of Fertility and Birth.* London: Academic Press, 1982.

Macklin, Ruth. "Artificial Means of Reproduction and Our Understanding of the Family." *Hastings Center Report* (January/February 1991): 5–11.

———. "Is There Anything Wrong with Surrogate Motherhood? An Ethical Analysis." *Law, Medicine and Health Care* 16/1–2 (Spring 1988): 57–64.

Mahoney, Joan. "An Essay on Surrogacy and Feminist Thought." *Law, Medicine and Health Care* 16/1–2 (Spring 1988): 81–88.

Malter, Henry E., and Jacques Cohen. "Partial Zona Dissection of the Human Oocyte: A Nontraumatic Method Using Micromanipulation to Assist Zona Pellucida Penetration." *Fertility and Sterility* 51/1 (January 1989): 139–48.

Marwick, Charles. "Artificial Insemination Faces Regulation, Testing of Donor Semen, Other Measures." *Journal of the American Medical Association* 260/10 (September 9, 1991): 1339–40.

Marx, Jean L. "Gene Therapy: So Near and Yet So Far Away." *Science* 232 (May 16, 1986): 824–25.

Mascola, Laurene, and Mary E. Guinan. "Screening to Reduce Transmission of Sexually Transmitted Diseases in Semen Used for Artificial Insemination." *New England Journal of Medicine* 314/21 (May 22, 1986): 1354–59.

McCarthy, Donald. "Ethics and Embryo Rights." *Origins* 14/11 (1984–85): 174–76.

McCormick, Richard A. "Document Is Unpersuasive." *Health Progress* 68 (July/ August 1987): 53–55.

———. *How Brave a New World? Dilemmas in Bioethics.* Washington: Georgetown University Press, 1981.

———. "Theology and Bioethics." *Hastings Center Report* (March/April 1989): 5–10.

———. "Therapy or Tampering? The Ethics of Reproductive Technology." *America* (December 7, 1985): 396–403.

McCranie, Martha. "Normal Problems in Adapting to Adoption." *Journal of the Medical Association of Georgia* 54 (July 1965): 247–51.

McDowell, Janet Dickey. "Ethical Implications of In Vitro Fertilization." *The Christian Century* 100/30 (October 1983): 936–38.

McGuire, Maureen, and Nancy J. Alexander. "Artificial Insemination of Single Women." *Fertility and Sterility* 43/2 (1985): 182–84.

McNeil, Maureen, Ian Varcoe, and Steven Yearley, eds. *The New Reproductive Technologies.* New York: St. Martin's Press, 1990.

Meezan, William, Sanford Katz, and Eva Manoff Russo. *Adoption without Agencies: A Study of Independent Adoptions.* New York: Child Welfare League of America, 1978.

Meggitt, Marie. "Humanizing Community Adoption and Donor Conception Practices." In *Proceedings of the Conference on Adoption and AID: Access to Information,* ed. Anna-Marie Cushan. Melbourne: Monash Centre for Human Bioethics, 1983.

Micioni, G., L. Jeker, M. Zeeb, and A. Campana. "Doubtful and Negative Psychological Indications for A.I.D. A Study of 835 Couples. Treatment Outcome in Couples with Doubtful Indication." *Journal of Psychosomatic Obstetrics and Gynaecology* 6/2 (1987): 89–99.

Mies, Maria. "'Why Do We Need All This?' A Call against Genetic Engineering and Reproductive Technology." *Women's Studies International Forum* 8/6 (1985): 553–60.

Miller, Steven L. "Surrogate Parenthood and Adoption Statutes: Can a Square Peg Fit into a Round Hole?" *Family Law Quarterly* 22/2 (Summer 1988): 199–212.

Milsom, Ian, and Per Bergman. "A Study of Parental Attitudes after Donor Insemination (AID)." *Acta Obstetrica et Gynecologica Scandinavica* 61 (1982): 125–28.

Milunsky, Aubrey, and George J. Annas, eds. *Genetics and the Law III.* New York: Plenum Press, 1985.

Mitchell, Lynn T. "The 1962 Kentucky Adoption Law." *Journal of Family Law* 3 (1963): 48–52.

Molloy, David, and John Hennessey. "The Regulation of Clinical Reproductive Medicine." In *Trends in Biomedical Regulation,* ed. Hiram Caton. Sydney, Australia: Butterworths, 1990.

Morreim, E. Haavi. "Conception and the Concept of Harm." *Journal of Medicine and Philosophy* 8 (1983): 137–57.

Murphy, Denise I. "Family Law: Rhode Island Establishes a Bifurcated Procedure for the Release of Sealed Adoption Records." *Suffolk University Law Review* 21/2 (Summer 1987): 397–404.

Murray, Thomas H. "The Gift of Life Must Always Remain a Gift." *Discover* 7/3 (March 1986): 90–92.

———. "Gifts of the Body and the Needs of Strangers." *Hastings Center Report* (April 1987): 30–38.

———. "Moral Obligations to the Not-Yet Born: The Fetus as Patient." *Ethical and Legal Issues in Perinatology* 14/2 (June 1987): 329–43.

National Committee for Adoption. *1989 Adoption Factbook.* Washington, 1989.

National Institutes of Health. "Newborn Screening for Sickle Cell Disease and

Other Hemoglobinopathies." Consensus Development Conference Statement 6/9. April 6–8, 1987.

———. Office of Medical Applications of Research. "Newborn Screening for Sickle Cell Disease and Other Hemoglobinopathies." *Journal of the American Medical Association* 258/9 (September 4, 1987): 1205–9.

Nelson, James B. *Embodiment: An Approach to Sexuality and Christian Theology*. Minneapolis: Augsburg, 1978.

New South Wales Law Reform Commission. "Artificial Conception Paper 3: Surrogate Motherhood." August 1988.

Newman, Lucile F. "Framing the Ethical Issues in New Reproductive Technologies." *Health Care for Women International* 8 (1987); 287–92.

Ng, Soon-Chye, et al. "Transfer of Human Sperm into the Perivitelline Space of Human Oocytes after Zona-Drilling or Zona-Puncture." *Fertility and Sterility* 52/1 (1989): 73–78.

Noddings, Nel. *Caring: A Feminine Approach to Ethics and Moral Education*. Berkeley: University of California Press, 1984.

Novak, Michael. "Buying & Selling Babies: Limitations on the Marketplace." *Commonweal* 114 (July 17, 1987): 406–7.

O'Connell, Laurence, J., et al. "Responses to the Vatican Document on Reproductive Technologies." *Health Progress* 68 (July–August 1987): 45–65.

Olsen, Frances E. "The Family and the Market: A Study of Ideology and Legal Reform." *Harvard Law Review* 96/7 (May 1983): 1497–1578.

O'Neill, Onora, and William Ruddick, eds. *Having Children: Philosophical and Legal Reflections on Parenthood*. New York: Oxford University Press, 1979.

Overduin, Daniel Ch. "'Test-Tube Conception': Some Ethical Reflections." *Concordia Journal* (November 1978): 244–45.

Ozar, David T. "The Case against Thawing Unused Frozen Embryos." *Hastings Center Report* (August 1985): 7–12.

Page, Edgar. "Donation, Surrogacy and Adoption." *Journal of Applied Philosophy* 2/2 (1985): 161–72.

Palm, M. Timothy. "Legal Implications of Artificial Conception: Making Babies Makes Law." *Medical Trial Technique Quarterly* 28 (Spring 1982): 404–23.

Pannor, Rueben, Annette Baran, and Arthur D. Sorosky. "Birth Parents Who Relinquished Babies for Adoption Revisited." *Family Process* 17 (September 1978): 329–37.

Parfit, Derek. *Reasons and Persons*. New York: Oxford University Press, 1986.

———. "Rights, Interests, and Possible People." In *Moral Problems in Medicine*, ed. Samuel Gorovitz. Englewood Cliffs, NJ: Prentice-Hall, 1976.

Parke, Ross D. *Fathers*. Cambridge: Harvard University Press, 1981.

Pellegrino, Edmund D., John Collins Harvey, and John P. Langan, eds. *Gift of Life: Catholic Scholars Respond to the Vatican Instruction*. Washington: Georgetown University Press, 1990.

Perone, Nicola. "Gamete Tubal Transfer as an Alternative to IVF-ET." *Contemporary OB/GYN* 32/6 (December 1988): 49–62.

Phillipson, Herbert E. "Adoption 'Plus.'" *Michigan Bar Journal* 67/6 (June 1988): 503.

Poland, M. L. "Reproductive Technology and Responsibility." *International Journal of Moral and Social Studies* 1/1 (Spring 1986): 63–76.

Pope John XXIII Medical-Moral Research and Education Center. *Reproductive Technologies, Marriage and the Church*. Braintree, MA: Pope John Center, 1988.

Posner, Richard A. *Economic Analysis of Law*. Boston: Little, Brown, 1977.

———. "The Ethics and Economics of Enforcing Contracts of Surrogate Motherhood." *Journal of Contemporary Health Law and Policy* 5 (1989): 21–31.

———. "The Regulation of the Market in Adoptions." *Boston University Law Review* 67 (1987): 59–72.

Post, Stephen G. "An Ethical Perspective on Caregiving in the Family." *Journal of Medical Humanities and Bioethics* 9/1 (Spring/Summer 1988): 6–16.
———. "Recent Works on Reproductive Technology." *Religious Studies Review* 15/3 (1989): 210–213.
Poteet, Gaye W., and Edie K. Lamar. "Artificial Insemination by Donor: Problems and Issues." *Health Care for Women International* 7 (1986): 391–99.
Quigley, Martin M., and Lori B. Andrews. "Human In Vitro Fertilization and the Law." *Fertility and Sterility* 42/3 (September 1984): 348–55.
Quinn, Warren. "Abortion: Identity and Loss." *Philosophy and Public Affairs* 13 (1984): 24–54.
Radin, Margaret Jane. "Market-Inalienability." *Harvard Law Review* 100/8 (June 1987): 1849–1937.
———. "Property and Personhood." *Stanford Law Review* 34 (May 1982): 957–1015.
Ramsey, Paul. *The Ethics of Fetal Research.* New Haven: Yale University Press, 1975.
———. *Fabricated Man.* New Haven: Yale University Press, 1970.
Ramsey, Paul, Stephen Toulmin, Marc Lappe, and John A. Robertson. "In Vitro Fertilization: Four Commentaries." *Hastings Center Report* 8/5 (October 1978): 7–17.
Rausch, Robert S. "Unwed Fathers and the Adoption Process." *William and Mary Law Review* 22 (Fall 1980): 85–140.
Rawlinson, Mary C. "Psychiatric Discourse and the Feminine Voice." *Journal of Medicine and Philosophy* 7 (1982): 153–77.
Rawls, John. "The Independence of Moral Theory." *Proceedings and Addresses of the American Philosophical Association* XLVII (1974/1975): 5–22.
———. *A Theory of Justice.* Cambridge: Harvard University Press, 1971.
Richardson, Jarrett. "The Role of a Psychiatric Consultant to an Artificial Insemination Donor Program." *Psychiatric Annals* 17/2 (February 1987): 101–5.
Riga, Peter J. "The Vatican's Instruction of Human Life." *Linacre Quarterly* 54/3 (August 1987): 16–21.
Robertson, Horace B., Jr. "Toward Rational Boundaries of Tort Liability for Injury to the Unborn: Prenatal Injuries, Preconception Injuries and Wrongful Life." *Duke Law Journal* (1978): 1401–57.
Robertson, John A. "Embryos, Families, and Procreative Liberty: The Legal Structure of the New Reproduction." *Southern California Law Review* 59 (1986): 942–1041.
———. "Ethical and Legal Issues in Cryopreservation of Human Embryos." *Fertility and Sterility* 47/3 (March 1987): 371–81.
———. "'Fetal Abuse': Should We Recognize It as a Crime?" *ABA Journal* (August 1989): 38–39.
———. "Fetal Tissue Transplants." *Washington University Law Quarterly* 66/3 (1988): 443–98.
———. "Genetic Alteration of Embryos: The Ethical Issues." In *Genetics and the Law III*, ed. Aubrey Milunsky and George Annas. New York: Plenum Press, 1985.
———. "Gestational Burdens and Fetal Status: Justifying *Roe v. Wade.*" *American Journal of Law and Medicine* 13/2–3 (1988): 189–212.
———. "In Vitro Conception and Harm to the Unborn." *Hastings Center Report* 8 (October 1978): 13–14.
———. "Legal Issues in Fetal Therapy." *Seminars in Perinatology* 9/2 (July 1985): 136–42.
———. "Legal Issues in Prenatal Therapy." *Clinical Obstetrics and Gynecology* 29/3 (September 1986): 603–11.
———. "Procreative Liberty and the Control of Conception, Pregnancy, and Childbirth." *Virginia Law Review* 69/3 (April 1983): 405–64.
———. "Procreative Liberty and the State's Burden of Proof in Regulating Noncoital Reproduction." *Law, Medicine and Health Care* 16/1–2 (Spring 1988): 18–26.

————. "The Right to Procreate and In Utero Fetal Therapy." *Journal of Legal Medicine* 3/3 (1982): 333–66.

————. "Rights, Symbolism, and Public Policy in Fetal Tissue Transplants." *Hastings Center Report* 18/6 (December 1988): 5–12.

————. "Surrogate Mothers: Not So Novel After All." *Hastings Center Report* (October 1983): 28–34.

————. "Technology and Motherhood: Legal and Ethical Issues in Human Egg Donation." *Case Western Reserve Law Review* 39/1 (1988–89): 1–38.

Rosenwaks, Zev. "Donor Eggs: Their Application in Modern Reproductive Technologies." *Fertility and Sterility* 47/6 (June 1987): 895–909.

Rosner, Fred, et al. "Ethical Considerations of Reproductive Technologies." *New York State Journal of Medicine* 87/7 (July 1987): 398–401.

Rothenberg, Karen H. "Baby M, the Surrogacy Contract, and the Health Care Professional: Unanswered Questions." *Law, Medicine and Health Care* 16/1–2 (Spring 1988): 113–20.

Rothman, Barbara Katz. "Motherhood: Beyond Patriarchy." *Nova Law Review* 13 (1989): 481–86.

————. "The Products of Conception: The Social Context of Reproductive Choices." *Journal of Medical Ethics* 11 (1985): 188–92.

————. *Recreating Motherhood: Ideology and Technology in a Patriarchal Society.* New York: W. W. Norton, 1989.

Rotunda, Ronald D., John E. Nowak, and J. Nelson Young. *Treatise on Constitutional Law: Substance and Procedure,* vol. 2. St. Paul, Minn.: West, 1986.

Rowland, Robyn. "A Child at Any Price? An Overview of Issues in the Use of the New Reproductive Technologies, and the Threat to Women." *Women's Studies International Forum* 8/6 (1985): 539–46.

————. "Women as Living Laboratories: The New Reproductive Technologies." In *The Trapped Woman: Catch-22 in Deviance and Control,* ed. Josefina Figueira-McDonough and Rosemary C. Sarri, pp. 81–111. Newbury Park: Sage, 1987.

Rowley, Peter T. "Genetic Screening: Marvel or Menace?" *Science* 225 (July 13, 1984): 138–44.

Ruddick, Sara. *Maternal Thinking: Toward a Politics of Peace.* Boston: Beacon Press, 1989.

Russell, Diana E. H. *The Secret Trauma: Incest in the Lives of Girls and Women.* New York: Basic Books, 1986.

Ryan, Kenneth J. "Ethical Issues in Reproductive Endocrinology and Infertility." *American Journal of Obstetrics and Gynecology* 160/6 (June 1989): 1415–17.

Rynearson, Edward K. "Relinquishment and Its Maternal Complications: A Preliminary Study." *American Journal of Psychiatry* 139 (1982): 338–40.

Sants, H. J. "Genealogical Bewilderment in Children with Substitute Parents." *British Journal of Medical Psychology* 37 (1964): 133–41.

Sapp, Susan Kubert. "Notice of Relinquishment: The Key to Protecting the Rights of Unwed Fathers and Adoptive Parents." *Nebraska Law Review* 67 (1988): 383–407.

Sathananthan, A. H., et al. "Human Micro-insemination by Injection of Single or Multiple Sperm: Ultrastructure." *Human Reproduction* 4/5 (1989): 574–83.

Sattaur, Omar. "New Conception Threatened by Old Morality." *New Scientist* 103 (September 1984): 12–17.

Sawicki, Stephen. "The Amazing In Vitro Man." *Cleveland* 17/6 (June 1988).

Scarlett, B. F. "The Moral Status of Embryos." *Journal of Medical Ethics* 2 (1984): 79–81.

Schenker, Joseph G., and David A. Frenkel. "Medico-Legal Aspects of In Vitro Fertilization and Embryo Transfer Practice." *Obstetrical and Gynecological Survey* 41/7 (1987): 405–13.

Schinfeld, Jay S., Thomas E. Elkins, and Carson M. Strong. "Ethical Considerations in the Management of Infertility." *Journal of Reproductive Medicine* 31/11 (November 1986): 1038–42.

Selling, Joseph A. "The Instruction on Respect for Life: II. Dealing with the Issues." *Louvain Studies* 12 (1987): 323–61.

Selva, J., et al. "Genetic Screening for Artificial Insemination by Donor (AID): Results from a Study on 676 Semen Donors." *Clinical Genetics* 29 (1986): 389–96.

Seper, Cardinal Franjo. "Vatican Declaration on Abortion." *Origins* 4/25 (December 12, 1974): 387–92.

Shalev, Carmel. *Birth Power: The Case for Surrogacy.* New Haven: Yale University Press, 1989.

Shannon, Thomas A. "Test-Tube Babies." *New Catholic World* (July/August 1987): 158–62.

Shannon, Thomas A., and Lisa Sowle Cahill. *Religion and Artificial Reproduction: An Inquiry into the Vatican Instruction on Respect for Human Life in Its Origin and on the Dignity of Human Reproduction.* New York: Crossroad, 1988.

Shapira, Amos. "Normative Regulation of Reproductive Technologies in Israel." *Nova Law Review* 13 (1989): 609–24.

Shaw, Margery W. "Conditional Prospective Rights of the Fetus." *Journal of Legal Medicine* 5/1 (1984): 63–116.

Sherman, Rorie. "The Selling of Body Parts." *National Law Journal* 10/13 (December 7, 1987): 1, 32–33.

Shewmon, D. Alan, et al. "The Use of Anencephalic Infants as Organ Sources." *Journal of the American Medical Association* 261/12 (March 24/31, 1989): 1773–81.

Simanek, Susan E. "Adoption Records Reform: Impact on Adoptees." *Marquette Law Review* 67 (1983): 110–46.

Singer, Peter. "The Ethics of the Reproductive Revolution." *Annals of the New York Academy of Sciences* 442 (1985): 588–94.

———. "Making Laws on Making Babies." *Hastings Center Report* (August 1985): 5–6.

Singer, Peter, and Karen Dawson. "IVF Technology and the Argument from Potential." *Philosophy and Public Affairs* 17 (1988): 87–104.

Slovenko, Ralph. "Sperm Donation." *Medicine and Law* 5 (1986): 173–77.

Sly, Karen Marie. "Baby-Sitting Consideration: Surrogate Mother's Right to 'Rent Her Womb' for a Fee." *Gonzaga Law Review* 18 (1982/83): 539–65.

Smith, David H. "Wombs for Rent, Selves for Sale?" *Journal of Contemporary Health Law and Policy* 4 (1988): 23–36.

Smith, George P., II. "The Case of Baby M: Love's Labor Lost." *Law, Medicine and Health Care* 16/1–2 (Spring 1988): 121–25.

Smith, Lucinda Ann. "Artificial Insemination: Disclosure Issues." *Columbia Human Rights Law Review* 11 (1979): 87–101.

Sokoloff, Burton Z. "Alternative Methods of Reproduction: Effects on the Child." *Clinical Pediatrics* 26/1 (January 1987): 11–17.

Spallone, Patricia. *Beyond Conception.* London: Macmillan, 1989.

Spallone, Patricia, and Deborah Lynn Steinberg. *Made to Order.* Oxford: Pergamon Press, 1987.

Stack, Carol B. "Cultural Perspectives on Child Welfare." *Review of Law and Social Change* 12 (1983–84): 539–47.

Stanworth, Michelle, ed. *Reproductive Technologies: Gender, Motherhood and Medicine.* Minneapolis: University of Minnesota Press, 1987.

Steadman, Jennifer H., and Gillian Tennant McCloskey. "The Prospect of Surrogate Mothering: Clinical Concerns." *Canadian Journal of Psychiatry* 32/7 (October 1987): 545–50.

Steinbock, Bonnie. "Surrogate Motherhood as Prenatal Adoption." *Law, Medicine and Health Care* 16/1–2 (Spring 1988): 44–50.

Stewart, C. R., K. R. Daniels, and J. D. H. Boulnois. "The Development of a Psychosocial Approach to Artificial Insemination of Donor Sperm." *New Zealand Medical Journal* 95 (December 8, 1982): 853–56.

Sun, Marjorie. "FDA Draws Criticism on Prenatal Test." *Science* 221 (July 29, 1983): 440–42.

Tartanella, Paul J. "Sealed Adoption Records and the Constitutional Right of Privacy of the Natural Parent." *Rutgers Law Review* 34/3 (Spring 1982): 451–90.

Taub, Nadine. "Surrogacy: A Preferred Treatment for Infertility?" *Law, Medicine and Health Care* 16/1–2 (Spring 1988): 89–95.

Tauer, Carol A. "The Tradition of Probabilism and the Moral Status of the Early Embryo." *Theological Studies* 45 (1984): 3–33.

Tooley, Michael. *Abortion and Infanticide.* Oxford: Clarendon Press, 1983.

Troup, Stanley B. "Reproduction Technology: Cataloging the Criticisms (Part II). The Medical Views." *Ohio Medicine* 84/4 (April 1988): 298–302.

Tyler, J. P. P., K. J. Dobler, G. L. Driscoll, and G. J. Stewart. "The Impact of AIDS on Artificial Insemination by Donor." *Clinical Reproduction and Fertility* 4 (1986): 305–17.

Uniacke, Suzanne. "In Vitro Fertilization and the Right to Reproduce." *Bioethics* 1/3 (1987): 241–54.

U.S. Congress. Office of Technology Assessment. *Artificial Insemination Practice in the United States: Summary of a 1987 Survey.* Washington: Government Printing Office, 1988.

———. *Infertility: Medical and Social Choices, OTA-BA-358.* Washington: Government Printing Office, May 1988.

U.S. Department of Health and Human Services. Centers for Disease Control. *Abortion Surveillance.* May 1983. [Annual Summary 1979–80.]

U.S. Department of Health, Education, and Welfare. *Legislative Guides for the Termination of Parental Rights and Responsibilities and the Adoption of Children.* Washington: Government Printing Office, 1961.

———. National Commission for the Protection of Human Subjects of Biomedical and Behavioral Research. *Report and Recommendations: Research on the Fetus.* Washington: Government Printing Office, 1975.

Vacek, Edward V. "Notes on Moral Theology: Vatican Instruction on Reproductive Technology." *Theological Studies* 49 (1988): 114–15.

Wadlington, Walter J. "Baby M: Catalyst for Family Law Reform?" *Journal of Contemporary Health Law and Policy* 5 (1989): 1–20.

Walker, Andy, Sue Gregson, and Eileen McLaughlin. "Attitudes towards Donor Insemination: A Post-Warnock Survey." *Human Reproduction* 2/8 (1987): 745–50.

Walters, William A. W., and Peter Singer, eds. *Test-Tube Babies.* Melbourne: Oxford University Press, 1982.

Waltzer, Herbert. "Psychological and Legal Aspects of Artificial Insemination (AID): An Overview." *American Journal of Psychotherapy* 36/1 (January 1982): 91–102.

Warnock, Mary. "Do Human Cells Have Rights?" *Bioethics* 1/1 (1987): 1–14.

———. "The Good of the Child." *Bioethics* 1/2 (1987): 141–55.

Warren, Mary Anne. *Gendercide: The Implications of Sex Selection.* Totawa, NJ: Rowman and Allanheld, 1985.

Warshaw, Robin. "The American Way of Birth." *Ms.* (September 1984): 45–50, 130.

Weiss, Rick. "Forbidding Fruits of Fetal-Cell Research: Ethical Issues Raised by Promising Therapy." *Science News* 134 (November 5, 1988): 296–98.

Werhane, Patricia H. "Sandra Day O'Connor and the Justification of Abortion." *Theoretical Medicine* 5 (1984): 359–63.

Werpehowski, William. "The Pathos and Promise of Christian Ethics: A Study of the Abortion Debate." *Horizons* 12/2 (1985): 284–310.

White, Morton. *What Is and What Ought To Be Done: An Essay on Ethics and Epistemology.* New York: Oxford University Press, 1981.

Whiteford, Linda M., and Marilyn L. Poland. *New Approaches to Human Reproduction: Social and Ethical Dimensions.* Boulder, CO: Westview Press, 1989.

Whitten, Charles F. "Perspective from the National Association for Sickle Cell Disease." *Pediatrics* 83/5 (May 1989): 906–7.

Williams, Bernard. *Ethics and the Limits of Philosophy.* Cambridge: Harvard University Press, 1985.

Williams, David A., and Stuart H. Orkin. "Somatic Gene Therapy: Current Status and Future Prospects." *Journal of Clinical Investigation* 77 (April 1986): 1053–56.

Wilson, Peter J. *Man, the Promising Primate: The Conditions of Human Evolution.* New Haven: Yale University Press, 1980.

Winkler, Robin, and Margaret van Keppel. *Relinquishing Mothers in Adoption: Their Long-Term Adjustment.* Melbourne: Institute of Family Studies Monograph, No. 3, 1984.

Wood, C., B. Downing, A. Trounson, and P. Rogers. "Clinical Implications of Developments in In Vitro Fertilization." *British Medical Journal* 289 (October 1984): 978–81.

Young, Iris Marion. "Pregnant Embodiment: Subjectivity and Alienation." *Journal of Medicine and Philosophy* 9 (1984): 45–62.

Zaner, Richard M. "A Criticism of Moral Conservatism's View of In Vitro Fertilization and Embryo Transfer." *Perspectives in Biology and Medicine* 27/2 (Winter 1984): 200–212.

INDEX

Adoption: as alternative to reproductive technology, xx, 114–15, 119; compared to DI, 120–22; costs of, 123–24; current trends in, 122–25; psychological effects of, to relinquishing parents, 128–29; and race, 130–34; and "unwanted children," 125–28
Adoption Factbook, 147n.6
AFS (American Fertility Society), 29, 47–48
AIH (Artificial Insemination Husband): and the Catholic Church, 4–9; and disembodiment, 5–6, 7, 8, 13, 17–20; and feminist opposition to reproductive technology, 14, 15; and natural law, 6–13
Allen, Charlotte Low, 147n.17
American College of Obstetricians and Gynecologists, 29
Andolsen, Barbara, 143n.11
Andrews, Lori, 80, 102
Annas, George, 85, 111

Baby M, 99, 101, 103
Baran, Annette, 85–89, 94
Bartholet, Elizabeth, 133, 147n.24, 147n.27, 147n.29
Bayles, Michael, 75, 143n.8
Beauvoir, Simone de, 37
Bhimji, Shabir, 145n.1
Blackmun, Justice Harry, 59, 142n.30
Bok, Sisela, 86, 144n.32
Bongso, Ariff, 140n.35
Bowal, Peter, 145n.3
Brennan, Justice William, 49
Brodzinsky, David, 145n.46
Brown, Louise, 28
Burnell, George, 127–28
Burtchaell, James Tunstead, 81, 90, 143n.2, 145n.48

Caesarean sections, 33
Caffara, Msgr. Carlo, 140n.32
Cahill, Lisa Sowle, 8, 79–83, 140n.33, 146n.29
Callahan, Sidney C., 137n.3, 144n.20
Campbell, Lee, 127–28
Capron, Alexander M., 100, 145n.7
Carey, B. E., 141n.9
Catholic Church, xviii, 4, 7, 9–11, 17–18, 26, 73. *See also* Vatican Instruction
Congregation for the Doctrine of Faith, 138n.23. *See also* Vatican Instruction
Children: as commodities, xiii–xiv, 8, 15, 19, 21–22, 54–55, 66; and experimentation, 40–41

Coercion: and adoption, xx, 126–29; arguments about, assessed, 35–40; and feminist objections to, 17; and IVF, 31; and liberal individualism, 32; types of, xiv, 32
Contraception. See *Humanae Vitae*
Corea, Gena, 14, 36, 140n.37
Crowe, Christine, 36–37
CWLA (Child Welfare League of America), 130–33

Daniels, Ken R., 85, 144n.25, 144n.30
Daniels, Norman, 137n.11
Davis, Mary Sue and Junior, 46–48, 51, 142n.8, 143n.36
Davis, Nancy Ann, 21–22
Deykin, Eva, 127–28
DI (Artificial Insemination Donor): and adultery, xviii, 90–91; compared to IVF with donor eggs, 96; compared to surrogacy, xix–xx, 98–103, 108; and the Catholic Church, 73, 90, 91; and embodiment, 75; harm to children, 91–94; and IVF with donor eggs, 95–96; and the problem of asymmetry, 89–91; and the problem of secrecy, 84–89; psychological studies of, 92–94; and self-identity, 93
Direcks, Anita, 28–29
Donchin, Anne, 139n.31
Dorfman, A., 141n.4
Dostoevsky, Fyodor, 71
Dworkin, Gerald, 137n.8

Egg donation. *See* IVF with donor eggs
Eisenstadt v. Baird, 49
Embryos: adoption of, 45, 67; experimentation on, 45; flushing of, 16, 18; cryopreservation of, 44–45; legal status of frozen, 45–48; moral status of, 61–62. *See also* preembryos
Engelhardt, H. Tristram, Jr., xvii
Evans, M. I., 141n.4
Experience: appeals to, explained, xiii–xviii

FINRRAGE (Feminist International Network of Resistance to Reproductive and Genetic Engineering), 5, 14, 18, 30, 139n.22
Firestone, Shulamith, 17, 139n.22, 139n.31
Fourteenth Amendment, 99

Genealogical Bewilderment, 93–94
Genetic engineering, 15–16, 23, 38–39
Gill, Owen, 147n.31

165

PAUL LAURITZEN is Associate Professor of Religious Studies at John Carroll University and author of *Religious Belief and Emotional Transformation: A Light in the Heart.*